Our Man SAM

Making the Most Out of Life with Muscular Dystrophy

Susan Bayle

Copyright 1998 by Bayle, Susan

Published by Susan Bayle, 424 W. Johnson Road, Scottville, Michigan 49454

Publisher's Cataloging-in-Publication Data
Bayle, Susan
   Our man sam/Susan Bayle
   Scottville, Mich., Susan Bayle, 1998
        p.   cm.   ill.
    ISBN 0-9667440-1-2
    1. Biography–United States.
       98-072339
       CIP

PROJECT COORDINATION BY BOOKABILITY, INC.

01 00 99 ◆ 5 4 3 2 1

Printed in the United States of America

DEDICATED TO:

Sam Bayle; All of Jerry's kids, their families and friends. This story is about a courageous and independent young man who had Duchenne Muscular Dystrophy. My purpose in writing this is to relate how we learned to live and cope with this disease; how important it was to pull together; how Sam lived his life to the fullest, enjoying each day and doing as much as possible! Along the way, I will mention some of the methods and improvisations we used to make our lives a little easier.

Can you imagine yourself being in a situation where you have to make the ultimate choice; To Live or to Die? To live awhile longer on life support or to say no more. Probably every day someone is faced with this dilemma, and this story is about how a 22-year-old man's life developed to a point where such a decision had to be made. It started on the 8th day of May, 1967. Sam burst into our lives six weeks early, and he kept our attention from that day onward.

He was ready early, but because of a complication called Placenta Previa, Sam had to be delivered by an emergency Cesarean. It took the doctor ten minutes to get Sam to breathe. Doctors don't worry about the breathing for the first seven minutes, but after that they fear brain damage. Sam's doctors felt he might be slower to develop mentally or physically. Sam had to stay in the hospital until he was three weeks old, and the doctor would call me every day about his progress. It was a very frustrating time for me. One day Sam was doing very well and the next the doctor didn't give him much of a chance to survive. I believe we were meant to experience Sam's presence, because even with his many setbacks and different problems, he was a very determined and strong willed young person. Sam survived and grew to manhood. He touched every life he came in contact with, and I believe we who knew him learned about ourselves and experienced many things because of him.

By the time Sam came home from the hospital, the doctor decided he was doing very well. He wasn't sure how much, if any, slowness Sam would have and where the slowness would appear. Sam was also born with two thumbs on his right hand. I worried more about how he looked than how he might do mentally or physically. Humans are vain; we worry about how we look to others and what they might think about us.

Sam had an uneventful and normal infancy. The only thing different was that, because he had been a preemie, he ate every three hours. He was a little slow rolling over, and when he was learning to walk, if put into a playpen he seemed frustrated. He acted like he wanted to do more than his body was able to; he was happiest when he could get where he wanted to go as fast as he wanted. A walker seemed to be the answer.

When Sam was one year old he had his extra thumb removed and he was in the hospital for about a week. The surgery was not a major event, but it was a long week keeping him entertained and making sure the bandages stayed in place.

We adopted our daughter, Stacy, when she was nine weeks old, Sam was four years old and Tom, Sam's older brother, was six years old. We still had no idea that Sam had a serious problem. But because of the difficulty

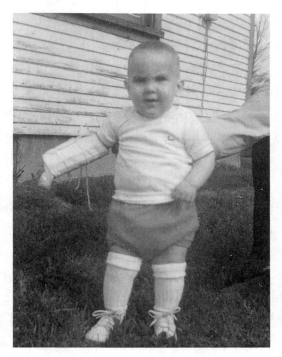

A big cast for a small area. Sam was recovering from removal of his extra thumb.

with Sam's birth, Howard, Sam's father, was afraid for me to have another child.

   Thinking back, I remember that Sam did walk, but he never ran.   When he entered school everything was basically normal. In fact Sam had a normal childhood. He could entertain himself for hours and loved playing outside, especially in the sandbox. When we were having our front porch built, for about a year it was just sand, not cement floor, and since it had a roof, Sam could play in the sand even if it rained. Tom was his father's shadow, but Sam didn't always follow their lead.   He was an independent thinker and doer. Sam did start having difficulty getting upstairs. Still, we assumed any physical slowness was due to his problems at birth. He would have to crawl up the steps, and to get down the stairs, he would go step to step on his butt. Howard got on Sam's case about the stairs, saying he was just lazy. Howard wanted him to work hard and help himself overcome his physical problem. When we discovered Sam really had a serious problem, Howard felt guilty.

Through the years, the pediatrician checked Sam's posture and coordination. He seemed to think everything was fine, given Sam's past history and problems experienced at birth. At the end of April in Sam's 2nd grade year, the Physical Education teacher was concerned about the many things Sam couldn't do in PE class. We took him to the pediatrician; it was May 8th, Sam's eighth birthday. The pediatrician checked him, and we discussed what might be causing him to have problems in PE class. He felt Sam might have a slight case of cerebral palsy, but with exercise and physical therapy he would be just fine. The doctor also ran some blood tests. One was the CPK test which tells whether or not a person has muscular dystrophy. I got a call later the same day; the hospital wanted to redo the blood test on Sam and also do a test on me to verify their findings. The doctor's office called me again after doing the tests the second time, and told me that Sam had muscular dystrophy. He was very sure that it was Duchenne's Muscular Dystrophy, which is the most severe childhood form of the disease. This type of dystrophy is carried through the mother. I was shocked, never having dreamt of such a problem The doctor told me to bring my husband to his office the next morning, and he would explain as much as he could about muscular dystrophy.

This was in 1975 and after trying to read the doctor's description of muscular dystrophy, I wrote the Michigan chapter and National chapter of the Muscular Dystrophy Association, MDA, for any information they had. I received one pamphlet about muscular dystrophy that described this disease: "<u>Muscular Dystrophy refers to a group of inherited diseases marked by progressive weakness and degeneration of the skeletal, or voluntary, muscles that control movement</u>." They have come a long way in this department; they now have pamphlets describing each type of neuromuscular disease. During the next few months I had several blood tests. Even as just a carrier, I had a very high count in my blood. They told me I might, as I got older, have a harder time using my upper arms and getting up out of chairs.

Within a week or two, the Genetic Clinic (Department of Human Development) from Michigan State University sent Sam to the Ingham Medical Hospital for a muscle biopsy. This would prove beyond a shadow of a doubt what kind of muscular dystrophy Sam had. We also went to genetic counseling and worked with a social worker. They were very helpful and understanding. The final diagnosis was Duchenne. The genetic counselor told us some facts we didn't know about Duchenne Muscular Dystrophy: 50% of all male children a carrier might have could have MD, and 50% of all female children a carrier might have could be carriers. After we got the final diagnosis, my sister took her two small children and herself to be tested. Sam's brother, Tom, wasn't showing any signs of the disease, but he went with my sister and her family to be tested. I was too nervous to take him. They all, including, Tom, tested negative. Because our daughter, Stacy, was adopted, we aren't sure about her yet, but she will be checked before having children. We could not trace muscular dystrophy back in my family, so the doctors called my being a carrier a spontaneous situation.

Howard had a difficult time accepting the diagnosis. It took him a long time to learn to deal with Sam's trouble. I don't mean he wasn't there for us, but he was having a hard time adjusting to the reality of the situation. The difference between how my husband and I dealt with the situation was communication. I would talk about the situation a lot, and that seemed to help immensely. We also learned a lot of families ended up in divorce trying to deal with the problems Sam had and would continue to have throughout his life. I was never blamed for Sam's problem, except maybe by myself, and my husband never gave me cause to doubt his love and support. One day Sam gave his dad a big hug and said, "Don't worry, Dad, we will be OK. We can get through this together." Howard went into the next room and broke down. I think this incident helped him begin to express his feelings.

After we learned Sam had muscular dystrophy, I went to school and explained to the kids and teachers what was going on. We also told many of our friends. Everyone gathered around and helped in every way they could. It was definitely an advantage to us to belong to a small and close knit group of friends and neighbors. The whole town was ready to help if necessary.

During the time we worked with a social worker and the genetics department of Michigan State University, they suggested we contact MDA, in Grand Rapids. This was the closest clinic for muscular dystrophy, but I was skeptical. I worried that this organization was just out to get our money, but finally called and went to the clinic at Blodgett Hospital. Dr. Puitt, a doctor at the clinic, impressed me with his knowledge and compassion. The many doctors and coordinators MDA has had over the years were always helpful, concerned, knowledgeable and very kind. I couldn't have been more wrong about anything than I was about the Muscular Dystrophy Association. During the first visit to the Blodgett MD Clinic, we were told most children with Duchenne's survive to the age of 20. After being told this, not one day went by that I didn't think about it. It was always in the back of my mind. It was a good thing that we didn't know about Sam's problem until he was 8 years old. I'm sure we would have babied him or felt sorry for him. As it was, we treated him like any other kid. When he got into trouble we disciplined him and if he did something good we praised him. I'm sure if we had known about his problem at birth, we would have worried more and not have let Sam just be a kid.

After we started going to the MDA clinic, they told us about the Jerry Lewis summer camp for people who have neuromuscular diseases. The first summer, by the time we knew all the details about Sam's illness, it was too late to register for camp. Camp is held each year the first or second week of June.

Howard played fast pitch softball for over 25 years. Many times during the summers the whole family would go out of town to watch Howard and his team play ball. For several years we camped when we went for a weekend. Almost every summer we spent at least one weekend at the Petosky State Park. We used a large tent with sleeping bags. The tent was plenty big for our family and we always had a great time. One summer that I can't forget was when Sam was about seven years old. One day Sam came walking back from the bathroom carrying his pants. He had on a hooded sweatshirt that was zipped up and from the waist down he had nothing on. All the campers around us were really chuckling and smiling while Sam came to our tent. Howard said "Gosh, I hope Sam keeps on walking and maybe no one will know he belongs to us." The toilets had been a little too high for him to reach, and he had had an accident. Sam wasn't even concerned about the picture he was creating, but just being a good kid and bringing his pants back.

That same summer we met and talked with another softball team. They were a much younger bunch of guys, but we had a great time with them. They really enjoyed our team's kids, played ball with them and went swimming with them. One of the young men was Brad VanPelt. He had just been drafted by the New York Giants and was very excited about that. He and his brothers also played softball every summer. Brad was flying high because of

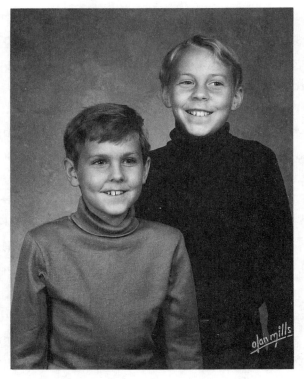

Sam and brother Tom, the "Dynamic Duo."

his NFL status, but made friends with all of us and showed us what a nice person he really was. After that summer, whenever we would see him he would make a special effort to visit with our family. The summer Brad found out about Sam's condition, he would go out of his way to visit with Sam. Brad was always concerned how Sam was doing and how he was feeling. They would discuss sports, especially the New York Giants schedule and how the team was doing and how they might improve.

Sam's 3rd grade went along about the same pace as 2nd grade. He did as much as he could in PE classes and his physical abilities remained the same.

Sam joined his brother's baseball team during the summers of 1975 and 1976. He couldn't get around very fast, but everyone gave him a chance to be part of the team. He had a couple of great summers.

When Sam was nine, we took a trip out west. I decided not to send him to camp, partly because of our trip and also because I was again a skeptic. You sometimes hear about kids being treated badly at camps and I just couldn't let him go. We took our trip to Wyoming and South Dakota during the summer of 1976. Sam was beginning to have difficulties walking, especially for any distance. We borrowed a wheelchair to use if needed. We rented a motor home and that was great. North of Casper, Wyoming, we stopped at a big ranch. During the trip Howard was also checking out Mule Deer hunting areas. We stopped at the first big ranch we saw to inquire about this and met Jack, the ranch foreman. I bet he was 65 if he was a day. He invited us down to his house and took us for a ride, about 60 miles, through all sorts of terrain, and all within the ranch boundaries. It was absolutely beautiful. He told us that part of the ranch was on the "Black and Tan Trail," which was a covered wagon trail used during the 1800's. This was the last trip Sam took before he went into the wheel chair full time.

Sam asked a lot of questions about his problem, but we were unable to answer because we didn't know that much about it, and we weren't able to find much information about muscular dystrophy. Sam was very interested in watching the Jerry Lewis Telethon over the Labor Day weekend. We learned quite a bit during that first telethon. One question came out of it that was a little hard to answer without sounding like gloom and doom. He turned to me, out of the blue, and asked, "Can I die from this disease?" I said that it was possible to die from muscular dystrophy, but also anyone could die tomorrow by just stepping in front of a car or could become sick and die. That seemed to satisfy him for a time. I always believed that you need to be as honest as possible with children; they are stronger than you might think and can learn to deal with whatever might develop in their lives. I was always willing to talk about anything and everything they might want to talk about.

Sam's 4th grade year was a very frustrating time. He would fall for no apparent reason and had a very difficult time getting up again. The children who didn't know what was happening to Sam were very mean. I don't mean physically, but they would tease him about the way he walked and the way he looked getting up from falling. Children with Duchenne's Muscular Dystrophy tend to waddle when they walk. Their chests stick out to help their balance and they walk on their toes. They have a difficult time getting up from the ground. I would describe it as climbing up their bodies. Putting hands on knees, then on their thighs, etc. Sam never complained; in fact, I never knew about the problems with the other kids picking on him until after the fact. Sam was very proud, and he didn't like asking for help, so he would try to do everything by himself. Mr. Spangler, Sam's teacher, gave Sam a lot of support and always had time for him. One very special thing happened because of Sam's condition.

There were two boys in Sam's class who were known as bullies. I believe Sam's situation made a big and important impression on the boys. I'm not sure why Dan and Scott became so protective. Maybe Sam was a little different and because they felt unaccepted by others, made themselves Sam's protector. Dan and Scott didn't feel sorry for Sam, but just accepted him as an equal. Over the years this was probably the most important thing to Sam, being treated as an equal.

In 1977, Sam was ten years old, the summer camp issue came up again. I was balking at the idea, but Sam insisted on going, so against my better judgement, I let him go. Again I was proven wrong for my fear. Summer camp was Sam's Favorite place in the whole world. The first time I took him to camp, we both cried when I left him. When I picked him up a week later, he cried for almost a full day because he wanted to stay longer. He always had a great time and hated for the week to be over. It also gave us (his family) a little time when we didn't have to worry about him every minute. Sam never had a bad counselor. They were always great, and the whole camp had a great time. They did everything possible. They had horseback riding, swimming, art and crafts, races, dances, camp fires and many more things. It was a one-on-one situation between the campers and counselors, and they became very close. I'm sure this is one of the reasons the same counselor and camper couldn't be teamed up more than one year. The counselors were usually college students.

MDA told us that as the time to be in a wheelchair

approached, something usually happens to bring the kids down for a short period, such as the flu, sprained ankle, etc. In Sam's case, it was a kidney infection. He was in bed for about three days, and that was the straw that broke the camel's back. During the next few months Sam had three consecutive kidney infections, and we were afraid he would have serious problems with this. But, as far as I know, he never had another kidney infection. Sam got his first wheelchair and he started physical therapy. This would help his remaining muscles stay strong and healthy for as long as possible. It would also help keep his heart and lungs to stay healthy longer.

Sam used the swimming pool at the Intermediate School District (ISD). He worked with the occupational therapist who helped Sam in many ways, mentally as well as physically. The wheelchair was wonderful for Sam, as his friends could take him with them wherever they went, and he didn't fall down all of the time. Sam had many spills out of the wheelchair because of the exuberance of his friends, but escaped serious mishap.

Around the time Sam first went into a wheelchair, we had gotten him a "Big Wheels." This is a kind of tricycle, but low to the ground. Stacy could easily push Sam on the Big Wheels and it could go a few more places than Sam's wheelchair. We lived on a farm on a dirt road, and the Big Wheels went easier on this terrain. Stacy would push Sam almost anywhere he wanted to go, they would go into the field and pick flowers or down the road 1/4 mile to visit their grandparents. They did a lot things together, like checking out cow pies and probably other

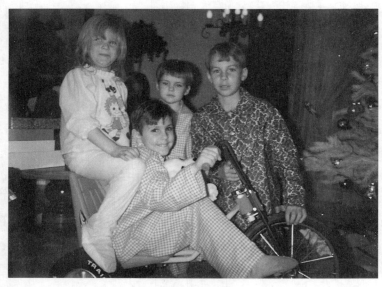

The "Big Wheels" was a great Christmas present. Also in the picture with Sam on board are Stacy, cousin Eric, Tom.

things I didn't know about. Sam and Stacy did their share of getting into trouble. They could each tell a different story with a straight face. You never knew positively who was telling the truth. It would make me extremely angry. Tom never was able to lie with a straight face.

Every year our barn cat had a litter of kittens in the milkhouse. Sam and Stacy would go down to the milkhouse every day to see the kittens. Well, one summer there was also a large bee hive located in the milk house wall, and every time the kids would go down to the barn they would see a few of these bees. The bees didn't bother them and the kids left the bees alone. One day while they were visiting the kittens, the wind blew the door shut very loudly and shook up the bees. All of a sudden Sam and Stacy came flying through the door yelling for help. The bees had become very agitated and starting flying after and stinging them. The kids were scared to death. I was sun bathing in the yard and didn't have any shoes or other clothes to protect myself while trying to help Sam and Stacy. Luckily for us, Tom happened to be in the yard and ran down and pushed Sam out of the way of the bees. Stacy had helped Sam out of the milkhouse, but then ran to save herself. From that day forward neither Sam or Stacy could tolerate bees; if they saw even one they would panic. Stacy hates bees to this day.

I worked for the school district as a school bus driver, so I was in a position to help Sam to go on all of his field trips. There would have been many times he wouldn't have been able to go if I or someone else couldn't have gone along to help. Another thing I was determined to do was make sure Sam could stay in public school. About this time the state was making laws that would allow physically handicapped children to stay in public school, and I was determined this would happen for Sam. Luckily for us and our school, a new middle school was built before Sam entered 6th grade, and it was all ground level. The law states that the schools must be handicapped accessible. Until two years prior to Sam's entering 6th grade, the middle school was a two story building. It would have cost a lot of money and hassle to make the old building handicapped accessible.

At this time, we had to start looking into how we could make our home handicapped accessible and also our best idea for handicapped transportation. Because we had three or four steps to get into the house, we decided our first priority was a ramp. MDA bought materials for the ramp and would have built the ramp, but because Howard could do the work, it saved time and money. When we started to build our ramp, we noticed something I bet none of us even give a thought to until or unless we have to: a majority of our homes are built with at least one or two steps up from the entrance. This is not a big deal until you need to maneuver a wheelchair. This caused us to obtain a set of two portable ramps that we could carry with us in the van. The ramps extended to cover up to three or four steps and this helped get Sam into most places he wanted to go. We also invested in an older van to see if this was the way we wanted to go for transportation. MDA bought us a fold-up ramp to use in the van. It did the trick, but we always had to have two people around when we loaded and unloaded Sam.

Our bedrooms were all on the second floor, and when Sam became too heavy to carry up to bed, we made our enclosed side porch into a bedroom. It was a small room, long and narrow. Howard cut a twin bed frame a little shorter and placed it across the end of the room. We made him a closet, put a dresser in the room, built shelves, and there was wall space to put his pictures. One important thing about the room was that there were plenty of windows and a door to the outside. I felt much better because there was an outside door, so in case of fire I had a way to get him out. Sam enjoyed his room. He could go and listen to his music or watch his TV. He put posters and pictures on the walls. He liked having his own space and to be able to do his own thing.

We also added a family room on the back of our

house. The family room was built on ground level. The rest of the house was up at least four steps. Because of the ramp, Sam could get into the rest of the house through the living room or his bedroom. To get into the family room, we either went through the rest of the house and down four steps, or came into the room from the ground floor. Sam could sit at the top of the steps (with large archway), talk to and see anyone who was in the family room, or he could go down the ramp and come into the family room from the ground floor entrance. From this time forward we heated our house with wood. That scared me a little. I worried that Sam and the stove were downstairs while the rest of us were upstairs. One of us checked the fire at least once during the night and when Sam became weaker and not able to move in bed without help, we bought him an intercom. All he needed to do was push a button with his finger to let us know if he needed help. The first time he tried it, it startled me so badly I almost fell out of bed. The intercom was also very helpful in getting our attention when Sam needed to roll over in bed. As time progressed he needed help more often, rolling over during the night.

Middle school, 6th grade, is quite different than elementary, but everyone accepted Sam very easily when he entered 6th grade. He had the same problems as other 6th graders: grades, homework, trouble in class, teasing girls etc. Besides, this was the first time the kids went to a different classroom and teacher for each class. It was a big adjustment. Sam was a B-C student throughout his school career. He was just like me - work like crazy and still get a "B".

Sam used a small table instead of a desk in the classrooms. He never lacked for people wanting to push his wheelchair to classes. The school waived Sam's physical education classes. He was still riding with me on the school bus. I carried him onto the bus and folded his wheelchair and put him in the first seat. Another driver took him home in the afternoon until he became too heavy to handle. Sam dealt with his situation with dignity. After he became too big to handle comfortably, one of our Intermediate School District's wheelchair accessible busses would pick him up and drop him off daily. A couple of incidents took place in connection with this arrangement. One was during the winter when the bus driver slid into the corner of our house. Part of the siding and the corner of our house went with the bus. Another was when our husky dog wouldn't let the bus driver put Sam on the bus. He kept putting his body between the driver and Sam. It was nice to know he was taking care of Sam, but the driver was nervous. Sam called me and I had to tie up the dog.

Sam also started going twice a week to our ISD to use the pool. Doctors maintain that activity and exercise will keep the muscles, especially the heart and lungs, in better working order for a longer period of time. One of the problems kids with MD have is respiratory infections. When they have a regular routine of exercise and therapy, it helps them keep their respiratory systems in better working order and free from infections. I believe swimming in the ISD's pool benefited Sam because he never suffered with respiratory infections until the last few months of his life.

Our Man Sam

After Sam was in the wheelchair full time, his heels and calf muscles started to atrophy. His heels started to tighten and draw up; his feet couldn't lay flat. The MDA clinic prescribed braces to wear inside his regular shoes or tennis shoes. The braces looked like a big shoe horn. They were made out of plastic material that was fitted and went from the bottom of the foot and up the back of the heel and part way up the back of his leg. The braces were worn under his long pants so they were not noticeable to other people. The braces helped keep his feet in a normal position and also helped us to handle Sam easier. After Sam had been in a wheelchair for approximately two years, the doctors suggested surgery to lengthen the heel cords. They said it helped some kids stand and walk for a longer period of time. In Sam's case it was more for comfort, to keep his feet looking normal and to help us handle Sam more easily.

For Sam it turned out to be a physically painful decision. The recovery from the surgery was uncomfortable, but it really made a difference with his feet for a long time. After the surgery, Sam was in the hospital for a week. He had casts on both legs from his foot to below the knees. Sam's incisions were closed with staples rather than stitches. I was curious as to how the staples were inserted. The doctor said it is done just like you would staple paper together. They use staples after surgery because there is less infection than with regular stitches. When they removed Sam's staples, six weeks after his surgery, they used an instrument that looked like a big staple remover. It was a few months before we could

23

move and handle Sam's legs without causing him pain. After the surgery Sam still used braces, but the braces were built into his shoes. He was no longer able to use regular or tennis shoes, but because of long pants, he was less self-conscious about the braces.

Seventh grade was a frustrating time for Sam. This was the first year Sam's friends could start to play and compete in sports, especially football and basketball. He really would have given anything to compete also. We talked a lot about how he was feeling and we took him to as many events as we could. Once the season got started it seemed easier for him to accept. If there hadn't been any time in the past that brought to mind his true situation, this year certainly brought it to the forefront. He was still going to the ISD twice a week for swimming, and I believe the occupational therapist who worked with Sam also helped him deal with his feelings. Sam was going twice a year to Grand Rapids to the MDA clinic and the doctors were pleased that he was healthy with no serious respiratory problems.

Sam's favorite football team was the Dallas Cowboys. They played in Detroit when he was 12 years old. His friend Ron, who also liked Dallas, went with us to the game at the Silverdome. It has a section for wheelchairs; it is located about mid-field and about half way up from ground level. There were some Detroit fans around the boys and they teased back and forth. They had a great time. The bad thing was Dallas lost in the last seconds of game. Sam thought that was a bummer! Sam's Uncle Brian went to the game with us; he was a Detroit

Lion's fan. All the way home Sam and Uncle Brian made digs about each other's favorite team, especially when discussing the last few seconds of the game.

During the summer of 1980, several families took a day canoe trip. Howard and I took Sam with us. Sam sat in the middle and wore a safety vest. Halfway to our destination, I grabbed a limb and over we went. Sam said "Mom if you are going to do that again, I will have a spell." He was kidding, but I felt bad about scaring him, so I traded places with a more experienced person to ride in our canoe and I floated down the river in an inner tube. Later that summer, another mother and I took our kids camping in the federal park. We had camp fires, played cards, took walks and went to the beach. The kids made sand castles and played in Lake Michigan. It was a real task for us to get Sam to the lake. We used a blanket and dragged Sam over the beach sand. It was hard work, but Sam loved it.

Eighth grade went along about the same. Sam had no major problems or illnesses. I believe this year he got the idea that he wanted to coach basketball as a career. I felt this would be an almost impossible feat for him, but it gave him hope and a sense of fulfillment to at least be involved in his favorite sport.

Sam started high school in the fall of 1981. He was excited, but nervous about the change to a new school. Everyone was great and he had a lot of good times during his high school career. Just want to say Sam was part of the crowd. During lunch in the cafeteria students had a food fight. It was a good one. Sam came home that day and said a bowl of chili went flying by his head.

Sam was starting to have trouble using his hand and fingers. We purchased an electric typewriter with a light touch, so Sam could type his school papers. You could read his writing, but with the electric typewriter his papers looked much better. I remember how the night before the paper was due, Sam was typing. I was just like that in school, the night before a paper was due I was up late getting it typed.

By this time Sam had grown into a good-sized young man, and because he was getting too big to lift any more than necessary, it was difficult getting his hair cut at the barbershop. I started cutting his hair at home. Of course, they weren't the best haircuts in the world, but it saved a lot of hassle lifting Sam in and out of a barber chair. I also cut Tom's hair until I accidentally clipped his ear and he said no way was he taking another chance with me. Sam was stuck, but didn't seem to mind. The other place that was becoming difficult to handle was the dentist. For a while the dentist and I were able to put Sam into the dentist's chair. Later the dentist worked on Sam's teeth without getting him out of his wheelchair. It was more difficult for the dentist, but was much easier on Sam and me.

During the winter months it was becoming difficult for Sam to wear a winter coat. The winter coats were too bulky to wear while in the wheelchair; he couldn't sit up straight. Sam's great grandmother made him a wool cape. You could wrap the cape around Sam and his wheelchair at the same time. It certainly solved the problem in an ingenious fashion.

A friend of our family flies a small plane. He asked Sam if he would like to fly with him. Howard took Sam to the plane and sat him in it. They flew all over the area and even went over our house so we could see him. He really enjoyed the flight and talked about it for a long time. I am glad he experienced that, because he never got to fly on a commercial airline. (Handicapped people can fly commercially, but you need to make arrangements ahead of time.)

At the end of Sam's sophomore year, we and MDA decided Sam needed a electric wheelchair. I believe this was the major event in Sam's life. He was no longer dependent on other people every time he wanted to move or to go to another room. The first time he used the electric wheelchair outside was at one of Tom's high school baseball games. We were playing in Hart and Sam just took off and drove all over the area. He was so happy to have his own wheels (legs) and to be able to investigate surrounding area. I believe this one happening helped him become as independent as possible; he could be his own person. He didn't have to depend on anyone at school to push him to classes, get to the bus, go through the lunch line. He felt great!

Sam had two teachers who developed a valuable friendship with him. They treated him like any other young adult. Sam strived all of his life to be treated as an equal. He taught Mr. Shriver, his PE teacher, some card games. They played cards every day, and Sam must have taught Mr. Shriver well, because Sam could never beat him. That probably ticked Sam off, but he never stayed mad for long and I'm sure he got even. At home, we had gotten Sam Atari games that could be played on the TV screen. The game had hand controls and he got very good at the games. One Christmas, Mr. Shriver got him a new model hand control and that made Sam even better at the games.

Mr. Taranko was another teacher who was first rate with Sam. He was the Wood Shop teacher and one day Mr. Taranko and several other students lifted Sam, wheelchair and, all and set him in one of the school's showcases and wouldn't let Sam out until lunch. We got some pictures; everyone involved had a good time; it was wonderful for Sam. I'm sure Sam spouted quite a bit about the situation, but it made him feel part of the group. Mr. Shriver and Mr. Taranko also coached different sports, and they would discuss all kinds of sports with Sam. They consulted with Sam about the pros and cons and many different things they could do to improve each and every sport the school had.

A former coach/teacher, Mr. Kudwa, kept Sam's attitude toward coaching on a positive note. Mr. Kudwa was excellent with Sam. He knew as I did that Sam's coaching dream was almost impossible, but he talked about the good and bad of coaching and always had time for Sam even after he left our school district. At one time Mrs. Keenan, the Spanish teacher, was in a wheelchair because she had broken her leg. She and Sam would have wheelchair races in the halls. Sam had developed a good friendship with two girls from his class, and a special

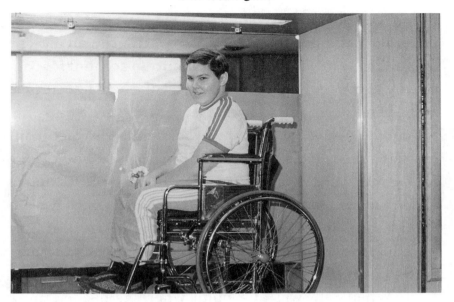

On display at the Mason County Central High School wood shop display case. Sam was out in time for lunch.

holiday never got by without one or both girls getting Sam a flower. Sam really enjoyed their friendship, which continued throughout his life.

Every year for Homecoming, Spirit Week, they would have some events that involved racing with bikes or wagons, anything with wheels. Sam always was in there somewhere helping his class win events in racing.

In the Spring of 1982 when Sam was 14, friends, businesses and organizations from our community had a benefit for Sam and our family. At the benefit, we couldn't believe the support we received from everyone. A band donated its time, food and beverages were donated, people made contributions and they had a huge auction. They auctioned everything from plants and beauty care to weekend get-a-ways. Some of the money he received from the benefit financed half of a Dodge van; we financed the other half. Benefit money also purchased an electric lift and the rest of the money went into an account for Sam for any needs that might arise. Everyone had a great time at the benefit and the van and electric lift were a blessing. My dad helped us save money by installing the electric lift himself. From that day onward one person could take Sam somewhere with the van. Before the electric lift, we had a fold-up ramp, but it took two people to push him up the ramp and into the van. The fold-up ramp worked very well, but there were not always two people handy when needed.

When Sam was at a point where he needed more turning during the night, we got him an eggcrate foam pad that fits on top of the mattress. It was more comfortable and the air could circulate around him and keep him from getting bedsores. We also discovered that a sheepskin was excellent for him to sit on every day. He didn't sweat as much, and it was very comfortable. My sister raised sheep and we had a sheepskin tanned. (You can also purchase them in stores.)

The kids were very good about helping with Sam. Anything that was needed was done by whoever got there first. For instance, my mother and dad recount an incident when Sam and Stacy stayed overnight with them. The wheelchair would not fit through their bedroom doors so Sam slept in the living room on a rollaway. Stacy was sleeping in the bedroom. Mom said she had fallen asleep in her chair and woke to see Stacy on Sam's bed bouncing and flipping him over. That was how Stacy was able to roll Sam over during the night. Mom couldn't figure out what was happening. Come to find out, Stacy had heard Sam ask for help in her room and Mom had never heard him, even being in the same room. Stacy was half-asleep, but just did what was needed.

About this time, through MDA, we were able to get a Hoyer lift. The Hoyer lift made it possible for one person to get Sam in and out of bed, the bathtub, or on and off the toilet. Before we had the lift, there always had to be two people at home to help him with these activities. The Hoyer lift also helped the people doing the lifting; it was getting to be as hard on the lifters and it was on Sam being lifted all the time. We were also able to get a sling with a hole in it, so that once Sam was on the toilet we didn't have to take him off the sling to take down his pants. The Hoyer lift was a godsend; I don't know how we managed without it!

In 1983 we added a larger bathroom. The old bathroom was made with a sink and counter top that Sam's wheelchair could fit under and he could use the sink to wash up and brush his teeth. It was getting extremely difficult for Sam to do these things with the old bathroom setup. In the new part, we installed a larger shower and the toilet was placed at a better angle that could accommodate Sam and the Hoyer lift with ease. About this time we also acquired a telephone speaker attachment. It was hard for Sam to lift the phone set, so with the attachment all he had to do was push a button and he could talk on the phone. He could do the same thing if he wanted to dial out. Neither Sam nor I would have been very comfortable if I couldn't reach Sam if necessary, especially when we started using wood heat. I was nervous about leaving Sam alone for any amount of time. We found a small fold-up table that Sam could use for his games and put the phone on. It was about the size of a TV tray, but was sturdier. One other gadget which helped Sam enjoy life was a 9" TV and radio combination. He loved to watch Monday night football but because most of us had to get up early in the mornings there was no one around late at night to put Sam to bed. With this little TV, we could put him to bed and he could still watch the whole game. It turned out to be a great idea.

We considered getting Sam a golf cart or something similar. He could have driven his wheelchair onto the cart and then used hand controls to move the cart. Sam could move easier on our dirt road and also go into the fields. We know a gentleman from Ludington who has a cart set up and it works well for him. He can take himself anywhere he wants to go. We never followed through on this plan because we moved to Grand Rapids. But, I feel it could be a worthy consideration for anyone who might need help with transportation for short distances and dirt roads.

A friend of ours who played softball with Howard worked for our local radio station. He introduced Sam to Tommy Roy, a disc jockey from New York, who had originally lived in Mason County. Mr. Roy learned that Sam was interested in the Philadelphia Phillies and Dallas Cowboys. He sent Sam many momentos from each team (including autographs, rugs, pictures). Sam also received letters directly from the coaches of the Dallas Cowboys

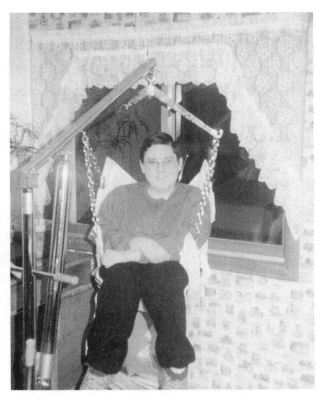

A big back saver, the Hoyer Lift.

"I didn't do it, honest!"

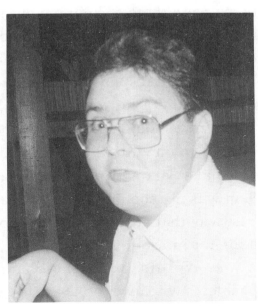

33

and the Philadelphia Phillies. During this time, Sam's cousin became a Dallas Cowboy cheerleader. She sent him signed posters. Sam's friends thought it was great that Sam was related to a cheerleader. She even stopped one time to see him in person. Boy, you can imagine how many of Sam's friends came to visit that day!

In February, 1984, Howard, Sam's father, passed away. Sam was a junior in high School. Howard had been sick and diagnosed with inoperable lung cancer in February of 1983. (Howard was 41 years old) The last four months of Howard's life he was in a lot of pain and was sharp with the kids. They had a hard time understanding and dealing with their dad. They knew he seemed mad because he didn't feel good, but they went through a lot of bad days. It was a very difficult time in our lives. His death made a big hole in our lives, but life goes on and we struggled forward. Tom graduated in May 1984. Tom and Stacy were there to help me with Sam, but his complete care was now up to me and I wouldn't have had it any other way. Tom had always been a stay-at-home kid, and I know he felt responsible for the rest of us. After Howard died, we did a lot of talking, at least I did, about what Tom's role should or should not be in our lives. I wanted Tom to go on with his life in whatever way he chose and not make Sam and me the primary factor in his future. Sam was my son and I would deal with the situation the best way that I could. Tom did go on to college and built a life for himself.

We did experience handicapped accessibility problems when we took Sam to the funeral home. There were no ramps or elevators, and we had a hard time getting Sam into the funeral home for the visitation and funeral. You normally wouldn't even think about such a thing, but we sure did at this time. Several people had to lift Sam and wheelchair (the wheelchair alone weighed 400 lbs) up and down several steps every time we went to funeral home. I suggested strongly to the funeral director that he make the funeral home handicapped accessible. I'm sure that we were not the first people who had needed that accessibility, nor will we be the last. Since that time, the funeral home has put in an elevator. This was just one more of many places we encountered with no handicapped accessibility. This was another important issue for Sam over the years.

The summer after Howard's death and Tom's graduation, Tom, Sam, Stacy and I took a trip to Washington D.C. Before our trip I wrote to get some literature about handicapped accessibility in D.C. According to the information, D.C. is supposed to be one of the best cities in the United Sates for handicapped accessibility. It wasn't too bad, but it wasn't great. A few examples: There is only one handicapped accessible elevator in the Capitol building and you have to get to it through the basement service entrance. The Jefferson Memorial has an elevator, but it was broken the day we were there; we had gotten a VIP tour at the White House and Sam had to use the president's elevator. One funny thing was everyone has to go through metal detectors and everytime Sam tried to go through, the buzzers would go off. The security people finally decided it was Sam's electric wheelchair that was responsible. We could get into many buildings, especially the museums and the Smithsonian Institute, but there were also quite a few places we could not get into because of the lack of accessibility. We stayed at a motel in West Virginia. There and at surrounding restaurants and stores, we found no handicapped accessibility. There were at least one or two steps to get over.

There were a couple of times we teased Sam, saying it was a good thing he was with us. One was in trying to find a parking place for the visit to the White House. Because of our handicapped parking sticker, a parking attendant waved us into a parking spot that was very close to the White House. Another was when we went to the Washington Monument; it was a hot day and the line went around the monument twice. When the guards saw Sam in the wheelchair, they took all of us to the front of the line and onto the elevator. It was a great trip and the last one we took as a family.

In July of 1984 Sam was invited to a MDA golf fundraiser through his uncle's company in Saginaw. ChiChi Rodriguez gave a demonstration of different golf shots. Sam had his picture taken with ChiChi and he was thrilled! The company also had a banquet in the evening and introduced Sam and other special guests. The whole event was great fun, and we met a lot of nice people.

In August of the year, 1984, Sam had back surgery. Kids with Duchenne develop Scoliosis, curvature of the spine, because they sit so much in wheelchairs. Until a few years ago patients were put into a body cast to stay

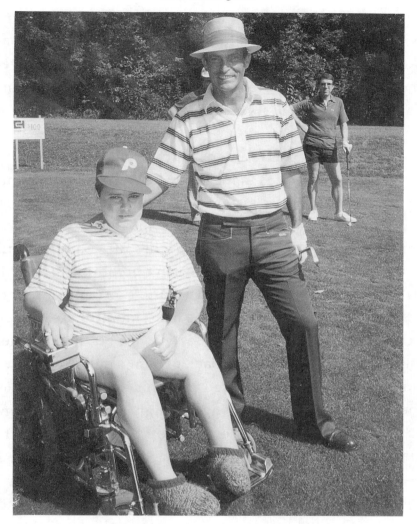

Sam & Chi Chi at a golf exhibition during the MDA Golf Benefit.

upright, which keeps heart, lungs and other organs from being crowded. The doctors now treat Duchenne patients as they would kids with a bad case of Scoliosis. They put an iron bar on each side of the spine. It is about an eight-hour surgery. Because of Howard's death in February, we, at least Sam and I, were leery and nervous about the

37

surgery. The doctors decided it was the best time in Sam's bone growth, so he had the surgery at this time. We had talked to another young man who had already received the surgery, and he eased our fear somewhat. Sam's surgery took about six hours and he came through it in good shape.

He was put into intensive care with tubes coming out from many places in his body; he was also hooked up to a heart monitor. I stayed with him until late the first night. The heart monitors are very sensitive and if something goes wrong, a buzzer goes off. Sam was still coming out of the anesthetic, wasn't breathing smoothly so the buzzer went off. This made Sam and me very nervous. Howard had been on a heart monitor the last few hours of his life; when the buzzer went off, he had died and I think this was in the back of Sam's and my mind. I finally had to leave because I couldn't stand the sound of the buzzer going off. During the night, Sam had become so nervous about the buzzer going off that he asked for the maintenance man to check the machine to make sure it was working correctly. The hospital understood Sam's concern and did everything they could to ease his mind. By the next morning Sam was doing much better and from that day forward the tubes kept coming out and he was well on the road to recovery.

We brought him home eight days later. It wasn't as painful to Sam as we thought it might be. I'm sure it might have been more painful if he had been walking and moving around more. The hospital didn't want me to bring Sam home without the use of an ambulance. They felt the trip was too long to sit up the whole way. My dad and I came up with a plan to transport him comfortably, and I was very determined to get Sam home as soon as possible. My dad built a stretcher-type gadget on wheels. We put egg cushion material on the part where Sam would be lying. It had straps to hold Sam in place while the car was moving or had to make any stops. We used pillows and blankets to prop him into a good comfortable position for the 100-mile trip.

Sam and I developed nicknames for each other. His name was "Whale" and mine was "Moose." Through the years we got good at giving each other digs while using our nicknames. Most people became concerned when they heard us. I think they thought we were mad at each other. We used the names a lot. In fact, one night after I put Sam to bed, I went and told him I was watching him on TV. He said "You are, what is going on"? I laughed and said "I'm watching Moby Dick." He said "Mom"!

Sam's senior year was probably his most memorable. During the basketball season, Sam kept stats for the team, was included in team meetings, wore a jersey and led the team onto the floor at each home game. He was able to earn a Varsity letter by keeping the basketball stats. He had no idea he was to receive a letter until the Sports banquet. Everybody stood up and cheered. It certainly brought tears to my eyes. Knowing the extent to which everyone appreciated Sam's presence was almost more than I could handle. At the end of the basketball season, Mr. Ingraham, the basketball coach, had a team party at his home and we were invited. It was first class.

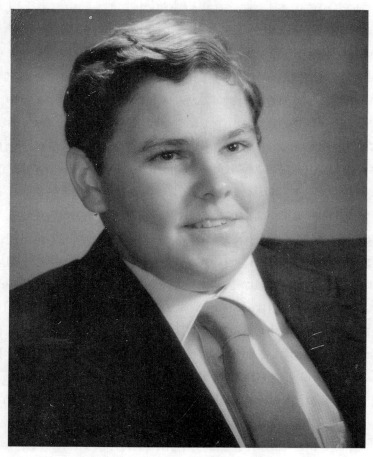
A formal side of Sam at his high school graduation.

Sam was chosen to be an honorary member of National Honor Society. The seniors also dedicated their yearbook to Sam. I talked him into going to his Senior prom. He said, "I don't have a date, I shouldn't go" and I said, "That is stupid; this prom is put on for all seniors, dates or not." He went and had an excellent time. He was chosen to be on King's court at the Prom. We got a wonderful picture of him and his friends.

I was able to surprise him at his graduation. I gave a speech thanking everyone for their love and support throughout Sam's school years. I think I embarrassed him but it was something that he would have done if he could have. And, of course I loved to surprise him whenever I could.

Sam started going to West Shore Community College in the fall of 1985. It worked out that I could take him to WSCC after I finished my first bus run in the a.m. or Tom could take him and bring him home after classes. Tom also went to the college.

I came home from work one day to find Sam bent over at his waist in his wheelchair. He had been in that position for about an hour. He had reached for something and couldn't get back up. He must have pulled some muscles because he hurt for a couple of days. After that I found a strap to tie around his shoulder and wheelchair to keep him up straight even if he reached for something. He was unhappy about the situation, but he understood he needed the strap. He was losing more independence and wasn't in control of doing things for himself.

In the Spring of 1986 I started looking for a job in Grand Rapids. I decided we needed something new and different to do. Both Sam and Stacy said OK. It was the hardest thing I ever had to do. I had always lived in the Scottville area, but we needed to expand our horizons and learn who we were. I got a job in May, and the kids were still in school. I came home on weekends until school was over for the summer.

It was hard for Stacy to adjust; Sam loved it from

day one. We lived in a handicapped accessible apartment. The apartment was on the ground floor. It had larger doorways, bathroom was large and wheelchairs could fit under the counter top and sink. Also the kitchen counters and sink were at a height for someone in a wheelchair to use. The apartment was in a large complex and there was a lot of pavement to drive on and that Sam liked. He was able to go on long walks even by himself. Stacy had come from a class of 90 students and went into a system with 350 to 500 per class, and she was very lost. We did enjoy all the things available such as shopping, restaurants, shows, etc. My folks also lived in the area, and we did a lot things with them. Our first apartment was brand new and huge. It was also within ten minutes of work, very handy. As time went on, I became very uncomfortable working anywhere too far for me to come home at lunchtime to check on Sam.

We went to the movies quite often. Every studio has an area where a wheelchair could park and the person could watch the movie comfortably. They didn't call them wheelchair areas, but we were able to find a flat spot to put Sam and wheelchair close to us. Tom was able to take Sam any time they wanted to go.

Sam enrolled into Calvin College in the Fall of 1986. It was the closest college to our home and without other transportation I had to take him to school and home. It turned out to be more than Sam could handle and after he had gone to school a couple of months, he decided he didn't want the stress. Part of the college was in an older building and had elevators. Sam was fine until he wanted to use the elevator without someone else also using it. He couldn't reach the controls. It was also getting harder for him to use his hands easily. For one of his classes he had to do a lot of writing and coloring, and it turned out to be very difficult for him. The last straw was when his own electric wheelchair broke and we had to borrow one from the MDA. The chair didn't fit him well, maybe just because he wasn't used to it; he was a little upset to begin with. It was his "late day" so he wasn't done until 5:00 p.m. When I got there to pick him up, I couldn't find him so I went looking for him. I found him sitting in a dark hallway. He was in tears. His borrowed wheelchair had blown a tire, and he had had to drive around campus with a flat tire. He had been stressed all day. Also no one had been around when he used the elevator. It had taken him a long time to get to the lobby.

He wrote me a letter that night saying he hoped I wasn't disappointed in him because he didn't want to continue school. In my mind the important reason for him to continue in school was that I didn't want him getting bored sitting at home all day. We talked about it and decided he wouldn't continue his schooling. We also talked about other options. One suggestion I had for him to was start writing about himself and his feelings, maybe at some future date he could write a story about it. This would also help get his feelings out and not keep things inside.

During Christmas of 1986, Tom and Sam drove to Florida to spend a week with my parents. Tom took on a big job taking Sam to Florida by himself and be on the road for two days. There was lot involved to care for Sam. Just for overnight they had to unload the Hoyer lift, a portable potty, battery charger and clothes. They had a fabulous trip and were able to visit tourist spots around Tampa. During the same time Stacy went to Florida with my sister and family. They spent two weeks visiting my folks and areas in Florida. Tom, Sam and Stacy felt bad leaving me alone in Grand Rapids over Christmas, but I enjoyed my time alone.

In 1987 Sam thought maybe he could find some sort of job that he could do. Sam got in contact with a department in Social Services that helps handicapped people get jobs. The lady he talked to was blind and that made Sam feel more comfortable working with her. We did find a bus that picked up people with physical handicaps and would take them almost anywhere in the city and surrounding area. He and I were real nervous the first time the bus picked him up. We weren't sure what kind of service it was or even if it was reliable. Sam was pretty proud of himself. He made the arrangements, went downtown, and came home all by himself. This gave him great confidence in himself. He was a proud young man and wanted to do as much as possible using his own devices.

After that he got involved in several things that required using the bus. The Department of Social Services worked with Sam several times. He never got a job, but it sure opened up a way of travel so he could come and go as much as he wanted. Through the social services office he came into contact with a group called Aid to Independent

Living (AIL). This was a small group who met at different times to discuss the many difficulties that come with being physically handicapped. This group had four or five people who were in wheelchairs. The group consisted of men and women with different ages and different reasons for being in wheelchairs. They had group meetings once a week and went out to eat lunch at least once a month. Sam really enjoyed it. He began learning how he could live on his own with a helper. He inquired into apartments that are government-subsidized housing. Everyone he called had a long waiting list.

He was so excited about trying to live on his own. I was so worried. I thought about the bad things that could happen. A helper who was mean might steal from or not take good care of him. I guess basically I was worried because he wouldn't be under my care. He really never knew how I felt; it was extremely important to him to be able to live as independently as possible. There weren't that many things he could do completely on his own. The idea kind of wore off when there were such long waiting lists. Being with the group AIL helped him be just one of the group. They talked about a lot of things that bothered them and some suggestions about how to do things more easily. Through this group, he ended up working on cable Channel 23 in Grand Rapids. They made him co-director and that was every Wednesday night. On this channel they had programs that were concerned with Aids to Independent Living.

Things were more difficult if Sam needed to leave during the day when everyone was gone. Quite often I came home from work to open the door for him, but I couldn't always do that. In our first apartment, we could leave the patio door ajar so Sam could push open the door with his wheelchair. Then he could close the door by pushing with his foot pedal on his wheelchair. Our second apartment did not have a patio or any door that opened outward. We tied a long strap on the inside doorknob, left door into the hall ajar so Sam could push open the door with his wheelchair. When he got into the hall he pulled the strap through the door. If he pulled hard enough he could shut the door tight and it would be locked. He then could shut the outside door with the foot pedal of his wheelchair.

During the summer of 1987, Sam assisted in coaching a women's professional football team. They were called the "Grand Rapids Carpenters". In the late spring of 1987 Sam was asked to represent MDA at a golf fundraiser. At this banquet we got talking to some people who worked with MDA. One girl there Sam knew from summer camp mentioned that Rahn Bentley coached a women's professional football team. Sam thought that sounded like fun, and the girl said, "Why don't you call Mr. Bentley? Maybe he could use some help with the team." Coach Bentley was also in a wheelchair and that in itself was a unique situation. The team practiced in Hudsonville, and Coach Bentley said, "Why not come to a practice the following week to watch and then decide whether or not you would like to be involved?"

Sam was excited about the team, so he joined in to help. The team practiced once or twice a week and played a game once a week, usually on the weekend. They did have a few games out of town, and we didn't make those. It was quite a distance to travel to Hudsonville for the practices so we made arrangements with the coach's sister, who played on the team, to pick Sam up on her way. Sam was put in charge of defense, and he just loved it. At one of the home games a lot of Sam's family came to watch. It was fun and everybody had a great time. It was a good feeling to watch Sam doing what he wanted to do most of his life, coaching! The team won the conference that year and, of course, Sam said it was because of the defense.

Sam was getting upset when he was riding in the van, because if we had to stop suddenly his feet would be jammed under the seat. Even when the wheelchair was in a locked position the chair would slide forward. When anyone took a corner a little quick, the wheelchair had a tendency to tilt one way or the other. When I invested in a newer van, we put in a new electric lift and safety restraints for Sam and the wheelchair. We had a harness and straps that locked the wheelchair into a position. It couldn't move and the harness kept Sam from falling forward. He felt much more secure. The company that put in the restraints said even if we rolled the van, Sam and wheelchair would stay put.

Sam's brother, Tom, got married in September 1988. Sam was asked to be the best man and Stacy was a bridesmaid. Sam was excited and proud to be in his brother's wedding. After the wedding the bridal party went on a trolley around Manistee and had pictures taken along the route. Sam was able to go along. At the

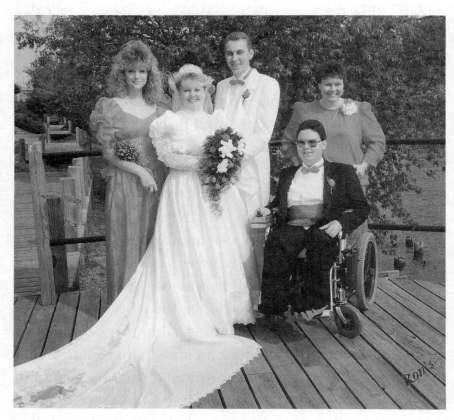

Best Man Sam at brother Tom's wedding with Stacy, Deb, Tom and Mom.

reception a marvelous time was had by all. We even have pictures of the Sam dancing with the maid of honor. It was the only time I saw Sam in a tux. I got some beautiful pictures. Tom and Deb lived in Grand Rapids for about a year, so they were closer to us and helped us when needed.

During the late fall of 1988, Sam had already turned 20 years old, I was unhappy with my job and it would have been my 25th wedding anniversary. I experienced emotional turmoil and cried at the drop of a hat. I was running scared. I knew that kids with Duchenne's had a

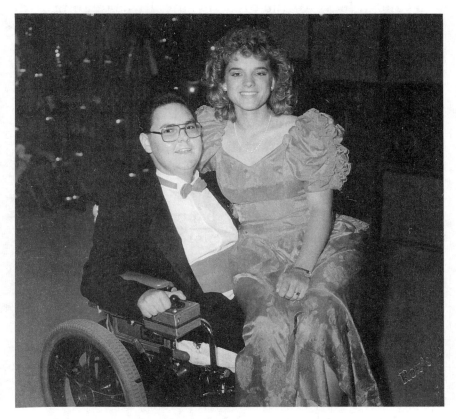

Best Man Sam and Maid of Honor dancing at the reception.

life expectancy of early 20s, I should have been able to celebrate my 25th anniversary and my job took me out of town daily and if Sam had needed me I wasn't available. I went to a woman's crisis center in Grand Rapids and talked to a counselor. I went back a couple of times and I did a lot of talking. It worked for me. The counselor told me part of my problem was I hadn't grieved Howard's death yet and I was already overwhelmed with the thought of Sam's death somewhere in the near future. Things finally started to straighten out in my life. Sam was fine, at least for the present time, I was dealing with Howard's death and I found a job where I could go home at lunch time to check on Sam. It comes down to either you learn to accept situations that come into your life or you don't.

During Christmas of 1988 my folks took Sam to Florida with them for two weeks. He had a fantastic time; the weather was perfect and Dad and Mom took him all over the area. Then early in 1989 Sam started having more trouble breathing. At first it happened at night and he needed to be rolled or turned more often. By March and April he would have small episodes even while he was sitting in his chair. The first part of May he had a really bad spell. I took him to the emergency room at Blodgett Hospital, where the MD clinic is held, and the only thing they could find was that his carbon dioxide count was higher than normal. They weren't really sure what was going on.

The next day I called MDA who suggested I take Sam to a respiratory specialist. MDA had an office of respiratory specialists to whom they referred MDA patients. During the time between making the appointment and the actual visit, Sam spent one night sitting up in his wheelchair. He sat by my bed and held my hand so I would know if he needed anything after I went to sleep. It is a scary thing to know there is nothing you can do if a person has problems breathing!

The specialist we saw was Dr. Katz. He appeared young and very quiet, but once we started talking to him, I was very comfortable with his knowledge. He explained

50

a little about what was happening to Sam. It sounded very scary and I was sure it was going to get worse. Dr. Katz and I realized that people who have MD don't usually get to the specialist level until the respiratory problem has progressed to a point where there is not much help for the patient. We talked about the future possibility of a turtle shell (a mini iron lung) that would help Sam clear his lungs of the carbon dioxide. A person breathes in oxygen and exhales carbon dioxide. When you can't clear your lungs, the CD builds up and you actually become asphyxiated. We also talked about being prepared to make a decision if the situation came to having to be on a machine to live.

Sam and I moved back to Mason County at the end of June. I had a hospital bed installed in the living room, and I slept on the couch. I thought we could adjust the bed so Sam could breathe easier and with less movement of his body. From the middle of May until the end of July I never slept a full night. I had to turn Sam at least once an hour. We got to the point where Sam would have little spells quite often. I wouldn't leave him home alone.

July 29th, 1989 will never be forgotten! It was a Friday and I needed to go to the grocery store. My son, Tom and his wife, Deb, were living with me, and I left it up to Deb to decide if she wanted to stay with Sam or go shopping. She voted to stay with Sam. I was gone about 1 1/2 hours, and when I got home I discovered that Sam had had a bad spell. It scared Deb half to death. She was alone with Sam when the spell started, and then Tom was there. It had been the worst spell that Sam had had. Tom really knew, for the first time, what we had tried to describe to him about the spells.

After I got home, Sam had started to feel better, but we discussed what had happened and what we wanted to do. We decided to call the ambulance. The ambulance and the fire department's First Responder arrived. They gave Sam oxygen, which helped him right away. It was going to be too difficult to transport Sam by ambulance, so I drove him to the hospital with the van. The ambulance and First Responder followed us and one fireman rode with us in case of problems. When we got to the hospital, Sam was checked out; the only thing they could find was a high carbon dioxide count. The doctor got in touch with Dr. Katz's office and Blodgett hospital who decided to have Sam come to Grand Rapids. We left about 10:30 p.m. to drive to Grand Rapids. My sister rode with Sam and me to Blodgett Hospital, where my folks were waiting for us. The doctors checked Sam over (I am glad Dad was there because the staff needed help picking Sam up and putting him on the emergency table). We arrived at the hospital about midnight; they did many tests and were also in contact with Dr. Katz's office. (Dr. Katz was out of town so we were dealing with another doctor from the same office, but he was unfamiliar with Sam's record). About 7:00 a.m. we were told that Dr. Katz's office thought we might as well head for home; they didn't think there was anything more they could do at this time. We got Sam dressed and were just about ready to leave when the doctor's office called again to say they decided to keep Sam for awhile. We were relieved because we had a real fear of going home and Sam having another spell. They put him in a sterile room (we had to wear masks); he was so-so all day. They would give him breathing treatments, but he didn't have much strength. That night Dad said he would stay with Sam so I could get some sleep. I didn't want to leave him alone. About 3:00 a.m. I got a phone call from Sam; he had gotten worse and the doctor had given him ten minutes to make a decision about being put on a ventilator. We had not had time to really discuss this matter - I told him to do what he felt was best for him. I went not knowing what decision he had made.

When I walked into his room Sam said, "I want to die." I believe at that point (after being wrestled around and put on a ventilator) there had been more pain to the procedure than he had anticipated and he was frustrated and scared. From this time on he couldn't talk. He was able to communicate by writing down on paper what he wanted to say. Tubes had been put through his nose into his lungs which blocked off his voice box (trachea). Because it was difficult to understand him, he would get very frustrated. I cornered the doctor and asked about the situation. I also said I wanted Sam to be able to make a decision, down the road, if necessary, about whether or not to stay on life support. At this time the doctor was very optimistic about weaning Sam off the ventilator, but also was understanding of my concern. This happened on Sunday morning. A lot of the family came to visit. We tried to get Sam in his wheelchair to sit up for awhile, but he was very uncomfortable. The next few days everything went along about the same. The doctor was still certain that Sam would be weaned off the ventilator.

Toward the end of the first week, I got a call in the middle of the night that Sam had congestive heart failure. Dad and I rushed to the hospital. They had given Sam some medication and were waiting for his high heart rate to get back to normal. It took awhile, but he finally was able to settle down and we went back home. The fast heart rate happened a couple of times. They were able to get the heart rate under control with medication.

The next thing he needed was a tube into his stomach to help him receive enough nourishment. The tube was put through his upper chest. I was able to watch this, as the minor surgery was done in his room. During this whole time they kept a close watch on his vital organs. The medication for the fluid was hard on his liver. One medication could affect one thing and then they would have to counteract it with something else that might affect some other organ. A vicious circle! Sam was getting upset with shots and pokes, tracheal tube, ventilator, etc.

The second week he developed pneumonia. Doctors became more concerned because the antibiotics needed had adverse effects on other parts of his body. They were getting concerned about his kidneys shutting down. The fact that he wasn't able to get up and move around also worked against him. On August 9th, Wednesday afternoon (my birthday), the doctor told Sam and me he needed to know in 24 hours whether or not to have the tracheal tube put surgically into his neck, which is a permanent situation. We started to discuss pros and cons (needless to say the hardest thing I had ever had to do-so far). I went out to my birthday supper with my family and told them what decision had to be made.

I was back at the hospital with Sam by 8:00 a.m. on August 10th. It was not a good day!! We discussed his situation until the middle of the afternoon. The doctor came in and asked how we were doing. Sam decided not to stay on the ventilator. His only concern seemed to be about me and whether people would think he was a coward because of his decision. I told him as far as I was concerned this was the bravest decision anyone would or could make. He was deciding about the quality of life he wanted to accept.

If he stayed on the ventilator, he would never be able to come home again, never be outside, and not be able to see his family and friends very often. He would have to be in a place where patients are on machines, a care home of sorts.

Sam decided against all this. He told the doctors he wanted to be taken off the ventilator. Toward evening the doctor came in and said, "I hate to ask this, but what time did we want to shut off the machine?" I didn't think things could be worse until then. It sounded stupid, like, "What time do you want to serve dinner?" Weird!! Sam's brother was going to be there soon, so we decided to wait until about 10:00 p.m. Tom and his wife, Deb, Stacy, my parents and I were there with him. Around 9:00 p.m. our minister from Scottville happened to come for a visit (not knowing the nature of our situation). Sam talked to him and I think Sam felt better about his choice, not that he was unsure about his decision, but the minister gave him just another positive understanding and opinion about his choice. All evening Sam talked about being in heaven and not having to be in a wheelchair; he also would be able to see his dad and great grandmother, two of his favorite people. He told his brother and sister if they didn't behave, he would send down a lightning bolt after them!

The plan was to shut down the ventilator gradually and at the same time to increase morphine, so he wouldn't have to struggle to breathe. We stood around his bed holding hands and talking to him. I was so upset I would have bolted out of the room, but it seemed that Sam would look right at me and I knew I couldn't (and didn't really want to) leave his side. If we had taken him off the machine suddenly he would have lasted about five to ten minutes, but he would have unconsciously struggled to breathe which had always been a scary thing.

Forty-five minutes later, the longest minutes of my life - he was gone. During that 45 minutes, he went in and out of consciousness and I believe he had several mini-strokes. His coloring became bad and it was just basically a terrible thing to have to watch anyone go through, especially a 22-year-old son.

Everyone was crying, family, friends, doctors and nurses. The hospital staff had been great the whole two weeks Sam had been in the Critical Care Unit. I received many cards from the hospital staff and Dr.Katz. Dr. Katz and I talked again about the possibility of his speaking to a group of parents and kids who have Duchenne Dystrophy about some of the things that could be in store for them, not to scare them, but to inform them. It might have helped us to know what could happen and to be more prepared to handle it. I believe we can handle things better if we understand them. Hardest to handle is the fear of the unknown. In fact, I believe if Sam had known what had been in store for him, the first time he was asked to be put on a ventilator, he would have said no. I know that sounds cold, but Sam went through a lot pain and discomfort for two weeks for the same ending.

STACY

What I remember most about Sam is his smile. I think if you asked people who knew Sam, most would agree that he was truly a happy person with a quirky sense of humor. Sam had a wonderful gift. He was able to see far beyond his wheelchair

A lot of people have a hard time seeing past a wheelchair. They forget someone is sitting in it. I have noticed that people either smile uncomfortably, or turn the other way to avoid a conversation. What do you say to a person in a wheelchair anyway? Well, a nice "hello" would be appreciated. After all, they are just as human as any other person. I realize that some people feel uncomfortable because they are afraid of saying something offensive. However, if you simply be yourself, things will turn out just fine. I think that's all Sam ever wanted to be loved and accepted and treated like anyone else.

I have also noticed that people seem afraid to touch someone in a wheelchair. I want to make one thing clear: everyone needs affection and love; this involves touching, whether it is a pat on the back, a squeeze of an arm and, yes, even a big hug.

Our Man Sam

Being Sam's sister was an honor and an experience I'll always treasure. I saw Sam, not the wheelchair. I spent a lot of time with my brother and hold on to each memory. We were good friends; buddies. As kids, we played together almost every day. Most of our summers were spent in the old red milk house playing with the kittens and secretly feeding the Hereford cows extra grain and hay. Sam would either sit in the old rusted wagon while I pulled him down the hill, or he would sit on his "Big Wheels" bicycle and I would push him. God only knows how I got him up and down the steps and hills by myself, since I was four years younger, but we always found a way to reach our destination.

Once reaching the famous milk house, the big challenge was crossing the barnyard, which was full of manure and bulls. This task was necessary if we were to find the spring litter of kittens. We bolted as fast as we could to get to the other side, hearts pounding wildly, holding our breath every step. We always sighed with relief afterwards and then laughed about the fascinations of cow manure along the way. Now the final excitement. Where were those kittens? I would climb in and out of most anywhere looking for them and reporting to Sam each find. We were hooked for the rest of the summer. These kittens would not be lonely.

One day after visiting the kittens, we slightly opened the milk house door so that I could push Sam from the rear. The wind took control of the door and slammed it against the exterior wall. Little did we know that two seconds later we would be defending ourselves against bumblebees. Yes indeed, there just happened to be a hive in that old wall. I instantly panicked and started to scream as bees were buzzing around my head violently. I still remember Sam's famous last words just before the sting: "Stand still and don't move and they won't sting ya." Well, just as I froze, a bee landed on my forearm and you guessed it; the bee stung hard. I never ran up the hill so fast and of course was crying and screaming the entire way. My mom comforted me and began making a white flour mixture to put on the sting, when she realized that Sam was still down the hill. Yes, I confess, I left him at the milk house to battle the bees alone. My mom sent my oldest brother Tom to rescue Sam, and from what I understand that was not an easy task. I assume the blast from the heavy door knocked their hive down, so they were not real happy with the circumstances. Poor Sam had bees buzzing in his hair and all around his body, but miraculously, he only was stung twice. Tom escaped without harm, but injured a few bees along the way back up the hill. At the time I really never realized how insensitive I was for forgetting to bring Sam with me up the hill. Today, I feel horrible knowing the dangerous situation I left Sam to overcome by himself. I am not sure why Tom was there that particular time and day, but thank God he was.

I consider myself very fortunate to have had so many wonderful memories of my childhood years with Sam. Because I was the "baby" in the family, I was not asked to help out with the chores on the farm like Tom. I would spend most of my time with Sam. I feel sorry for

Tom when I think about how hard it must have been for him knowing Sam and I were on another adventure while he was working his butt off in the fields. Tom really did not have as much freedom or opportunity to spend time with Sam as I did, which I am sure he resented me for. We did not get along very well at all, and with each day I am beginning to understand why. Tom spent long hours helping my father feed and count cattle, haul and spread manure, plant and harvest wheat and grains, and even cut and bail hay and straw. He would also help during the winter with the plowing of snow and gathering of wood. Tom was my father's right-hand-man.

While Tom was doing his farm duties, Sam and I were busy playing. I remember one day we decided to cover new territories, primarily after the horrifying experience with the bees. Rather than stopping at the milk house, I pushed Sam as quickly as I could up the hill to the pasture area. With 80 acres of land, we had a lot of ground to cover. Of course, with our fascination of feces, we made our way to the "cow pies." We created a disgusting game. As I pushed Sam on his hot wheels we would seek to find the biggest and freshest cow pie and run right through it, which eventually turned into a game of how dirty I could get mom's black rubber boots (I stomped in the cow pies). We were in hysterics with laughter. The reason I share this story with you is not to gross you out, but rather to point out that we were like any other brother and sister investigating all avenues of living on a farm. Nothing was going to get in our way. It did not matter that Sam was physically challenged. We were two determined kids who set out to accomplish anything that came our way. Whether it was jumping in and out of the garden and sewer in search of frogs and snakes, or taking a "walk" into town to buy candy at the local drugstore. If we wanted it, we were going to get it.

Wintertime was also fun for us. Tom took part in most of our winter activities. Living in Michigan, we had a lot of snowy days. King on the Mountain was a favorite game for us to play, but we also built forts out of large piles of snow that Dad or Grandpa had plowed, or just out of the large natural drifts. Because we lived on a large hill, we also had fun sledding. Tom was old enough to take us on the snowmobile, so Sam and I took turns riding with him.

I don't remember spending a lot of time with friends during my childhood - other than Sam. The only time that really comes to mind is when Sam started attending MDA Camp. He would go for about six days. I would either stay with my grandparents during this time or Mom would arrange for me to spend time at one of the local lakes with a girlfriend. I'm sure that Mom needed the time to herself and with my father.

While Sam was at MDA Camp in Holland, MI, he learned a lot of new games and activities. As soon as he returned home from camp, he told us of all the fun things he was able to participate in, such as bowling, whiffle ball, dancing, swimming, horseback riding, and relay races. A favorite of his was whiffle ball. I would pitch to Sam as he swung a bat at the ball. We both benefited from the sport. Sam exercised several different muscles throughout his body, and I became a pretty good pitcher. Dad caught on to this and practiced with me almost every day. I ended up pitching fast pitch softball for two years, but then learned new interests. I was also into basketball for a while. Sam used to help me practice by guarding me with his wheelchair. Once Sam obtained his electric wheelchair, this became a huge challenge and exhausting practice. Sam enjoyed sports, so he was a good advisor for me. My father was active in both softball and basketball as well, but unfortunately Dad died of lung cancer before my peak years, so he did not get much opportunity to work with me. Sports were introduced to us at an early age as my father played fast pitch softball every summer. Sam helped a lot with stats and score keeping for both softball and basketball. His dream was to become a coach.

I would go with Sam sometimes to the Intermediate Center where he would receive occupational therapy. I would mostly swim in the pool, but was aware of where Sam was at all times. I remember feeling upset a few times because I could tell Sam was hurting. I knew the therapist was tying to help Sam, but I was naturally protective. I think going to the Intermediate Center was when the reality that Sam was physically challenged hit me. I can remember sitting with my mother while she spoke to the therapist about the disease's progression. I was not sure of what all the words meant, but I knew that Sam was not improving. The realization of the disease scared me and I know that I started building walls around myself. I was confused about what was going to happen to my brother. Not only do we need to educate the person who is physically challenged, but it would be helpful if the entire family were knowledgeable about what could be expected. I remember my mother mentioning that at the time there wasn't a lot of literature. The more supportive groups, and the more doctors and nurses honestly communicating with all parties involved, the easier it will be for families to cope with this devastating disease. This disease, like all others, should be approached with a team attitude

As I became a teenager, and Sam was nearly finished with high school, we started getting involved with our own interests. Sam was active with sport affiliations and I was shifting interests from sports to more art-oriented activities such as band and drama. Of course boys were moving to the top of my list of priorities as well as spending time with classmates. I feel guilty now for not spending more time with Sam during those few years. Every moment is so precious.

Two years after my father died, Sam was graduated from high school and I had completed my freshman year. Mom moved us to the "Big City" of Grand Rapids. Tom stayed at the house with a buddy (the farm animals and equipment were sold after my father died). Mom returned to college to finish her degree, Sam took advantage of the accessibilities in the city and enrolled in college and later worked for a local television station, and I settled into a new school. I have some regrets about my high school years. I wish I had asked Sam to my prom because it would have been such an honor. We didn't show a lot of affection towards one another, so the thought never occurred to me. I wish I had invited Sam to the movies or even out to a nice dinner. He must have been lonely in Grand Rapids not knowing many people. I wonder if he ever wished I would ask him to join my friends and me. I feel I was insensitive for not including him. I suppose the only way I can excuse my ignorance is to understand the fact that I was a hormonal teenager adjusting to a new environment. I was not a very pleasant person to be around during this change, which I don't think family members understand, but they did not go through the same experiences I did with this move. I agree however, that though it was tough, it was beneficial for me in the long run.

My senior year was the most difficult time for me. As I started maturing, I started facing reality. Sam was getting older and weaker and I was running out of time with him. Around March of 1989 I started pulling away from my friends. Of course, my friends didn't know what was going on. Whenever they invited me to do something, I hesitated because I did not want to hurt Sam's feelings. I did not think it was fair that I could experience things that Sam could not experience. My friends started growing impatient with me as I drifted further and further away from them. I then started looking for a boyfriend because for some reason I felt that I wanted to get married right away so that Sam would have known my husband. Sounds silly for an eighteen-year-old, but when you're losing someone, strange thoughts go through your head. Thank God I woke up!

Sam started developing breathing problems. I remember starting to fall asleep a lot during my classes because I was worried at night that Sam was going to stop breathing. I would hear Sam calling for Mom or me to change his sleeping position, as he could not breathe correctly in his current position. The first time scared the hell out of me, as I did not understand what was happening,

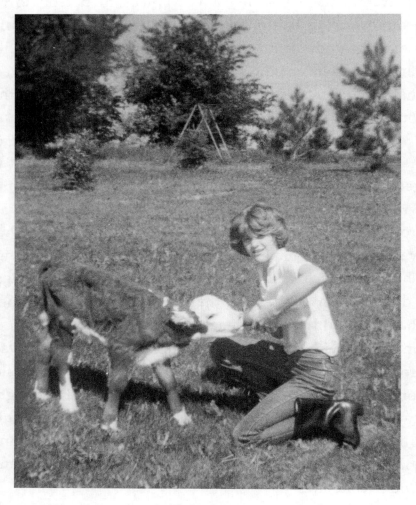

Stacy feeding a calf, a farm girl at work wearing the infamous black (cowpie) boots.

but with each recurrence, I faced reality. Sam was scared too because he did not know what would happen next. I can still see the fear and sadness in his eyes.

With Sam slowly slipping away, I started holding on as much as I could. Especially after my Mom shared with me that Sam and she were returning to the house on the farm after my graduation. Mom let me decide whether or not I wanted to go with them for the summer. At 18, I had just met "a guy" and had pushed away most of my friends. But I was planning to go off to college with my best friend the following fall. Being in denial about the circumstances of my brother, I chose to stay in Grand Rapids, with my grandparents until I left for college. I was fighting a lot with my mother and my friends were angry with me because they did not understand what I was going through. All I knew was I did not want to lose my boy friend too, so I did not want to move away from him.

It was never a hassle to me to help Sam with his needs. I remember many nights; especially after my father died, helping my mother lift Sam into or out of the bed or onto or off of the toilet. As I got older, I would bathe and dress him, help him with urinals, and even lift him to bed. We did not have the equipment to aid in these tasks until a benefit took place in Sam's honor. This benefit occurred at the town's Optimist Club, which many citizens attended and donated money to help Sam. From this benefit we were able to buy a van, install an electrical lift into the van, and thank goodness, provide a Hoyer lift to help lift Sam into and out of the shower and into and out of bed. I want to thank everyone for their generosity.

Transportation: people, if you are the driver of any vehicle transporting the physically challenged, please remember to drive carefully. Sam was flipped over a few times in his life which both scared and injured him.

I would also cook many meals for Sam, which I loved to do. Sam's all time favorite was macaroni & cheese and grilled cheese sandwiches. I became a pro at these items. Sam would help me sometimes too! I remember when we were just kids; we attempted to make my mother a birthday cake. Yes, I said attempt. It was a little runny, no matter how long we baked it, but the birds seemed to enjoy it.

By August 1989, I was still dating this guy and made several trips back home to visit. I was still planning to go to college with my best friend, even though we rarely saw each other. One night while at my grandparents with my boyfriend, I started to cry. Felt like something was wrong. Thirty minutes later, I received a phone call that my mother was bringing Sam to Grand Rapids because he needed medical attention. We went to the hospital to wait for them. When they arrived, they took Sam to an examination room. I remember my mom looking at me and saying, "What's wrong Stacy? It looks like you saw a ghost." I guess it scared me that I felt Sam's danger that night before I even knew that he was in trouble. I remember going into the examination room to see him and just wanting to take away his pain. He had suffered so much in the past six months. Sam had a horrible headache, so I sat next to him and massaged his head. It put him to sleep, but not for long. The doctor's had news for him. Sam was having an imbalance of CO2 and Oxygen, which was causing the headache and dizziness. They hospitalized him that night. He would never see the outside world again.

That evening my mother was awakened by a phone call from Sam. He was terrified because the doctors were asking him to choose whether or not to have a tracheotomy performed; placing him on a ventilator. It was the last time my mother ever heard his voice. He would not be able to speak again.

Sam had developed pneumonia and desperately needed help. He chose the ventilator. The rest of the story will follow in a brief essay I wrote for a class my freshman year of college:

THE FINAL DECISION

Can you imagine having to choose between life and death? Can you imagine having to choose a day and time to make that final decision?

My brother Sam was forced to make a decision on whether or not he was ready to go onward to another world which we call heaven or whether he wanted to suffer for the rest of his life.

Sam was born with Duchennes Muscular Dystrophy. Muscular Dystrophy is a fatal disease that breaks down your muscles over a period of time. The life span for most people with Duchennes ranges from late teens to early twenties. Sam was twenty-two. He had reached his final stages. Throughout the summer of 1989, Sam had developed a slight case of pneumonia.

The doctors were not the least bit concerned, but they had decided to admit him for one night for more testing. This frightened my family and me because we knew that this was the beginning of a long and emotional time for all of us. We always knew that someday something would happen, but on one can ever fully prepare themselves for someone's death.

After being admitted into the hospital for one night, Sam had called my mother and oldest brother Tom at three a.m. and told us he had to make a decision within the next five minutes to go on a life supporting machine or just let himself rest in peace. We knew he had to make the decision himself, but we all had been a little selfish and wanted him to remain with us. We immediately rushed to the hospital to be with him. When we had arrived, Sam had already chosen to go on the life support system.

My family and I were relieved that Sam had chosen to fight for his life. There was not a day that we did not spend with him because we wanted to make sure he knew we loved and cared for him and that we were behind him all the way.

After a long two weeks of going to visit my brother, my family and I began to grow sad. Watching a young and cheerful man suffer in the hospital, hooked up to several tubes and being constantly nursed was an awful sight to see. All of us knew Sam was unhappy. I can remember when Sam first got connected to the machine. He told us he wanted to die. The life support system was different than he expected. He was frustrated from the medications the nurses were giving him and he was sore from all of the tubes he had connected to his nose and his mouth. Most of all, Sam was very unhappy because he knew he would never be able to talk or go outside again.

Our Man Sam

On the date of August 10, 1989, Sam was faced with another major decision. He was not getting much rest because he was having problems breathing. Sam was beginning to take a turn for the worse. Sam's doctors introduced to him a tracheotomy. A tracheotomy is an incision of the trachea to aid breathing in case of an emergency. If he had decided to go with the trachea operation, it would be a matter of a few weeks, months, or years before his internal organs would begin to fail. He also had found out that even with the operation he still would not be able to talk to us.

After a long day of thinking, Sam made his final decision. He told us he was ready to move on. He said to us all: "I will be happy in heaven. There are no wheelchairs there and I will be able to play sports and be with Dad and Granny." After Sam had told us each his own personal message and spent the time with us he felt we needed, he notified the nurses and his doctor that he was ready.

As we all gathered around Sam's bed, praying with him and holding him and each other, the nurse gradually gave him more medication to ease his discomfort and turned down his oxygen one level at the same time. Sam slowly began to fall asleep, opening his eyes occasionally to be sure his family were all still with him. His breathing seemed to become very heavy and more rapid. He kept fighting to not fall asleep, but the medications overpowered his strength. Then the horror arrived.

At approximately 11:45 p.m., Sam looked at his brother and took his last breath. We all hesitated, waiting for him to gasp for another breath, but he had already past on. As I felt a part of Sam leave me, I almost let out a sigh of relief. I knew where he was and I knew all of his dreams could finally come *true. Though I was very somber and hurt that I would not see him for a long, long time, I knew that this was the best for him.*

Through this experience I have learned so much about life. I learned to live life to its fullest and to think more positively about life in general. Sam was a very brave and understanding brother and friend who touched a lot of people's hearts.

Sam Bayle will never be forgotten!

I ended up going to a different college than I had intended. Once my brother was hospitalized, I did some soul-searching. I had no idea what the near future entailed, but I knew that I was not going to leave Sam. He could have been in and out of the hospital one hundred times before he died, who knew? So, I made the ultimate decision to not go to the university with my best friend as planned. I canceled about three weeks before enrollment. I knew what was more important to me; my family. I wanted to pursue my education, but wanted to stay close to my brother. I spoke to Sam and my mother about my feelings and enrolled into a local college the next day. I remember visiting Sam after orientation and being so proud of myself. He was happy for me.

I started college about a week after Sam died. It was very difficult at times, but it was my best performance ever academically. I was depressed at times, but what helped me through it all was the fact that I knew Sam was still with me. In my heart, soul and mind. I have gone through probably every emotion since Sam died. Anger, regret, sadness, happiness, depression, etc. . . . Some people get angry with God. They blame God for taking people away. I was angry for a while, but then I realized that God does not punish. He rewards.

TOM'S THOUGHTS

There are many memories, good and bad, and I can't write about all of them. Here are a few that stick out in my mind. The best thing that happened for Sam was the electric wheelchair. What a lifesaver. Now Sam was free to go wherever he wanted. He could go for miles on a charge. Many times Sam would say "I'm going for a ride," and he might be gone for an hour or two. He could go to his classes at his own time and pace.

The electric wheelchair was Sam's freedom. He must have put a million miles on his first chair. That chair lasted several years. But they are also very expensive. Without MDA's help I don't know if we could have afforded an electric wheelchair.

Sam told me on many occasions that he would do anything to be able to play sports for one day. "Just one day." He said that would satisfy him. I knew that wasn't true, though. One day wouldn't have been enough.

He always said he could kick my butt in anything. I always replied "Yeah!Yeah!Yeah!!" So we would start going back and forth like two macho guys. Then it would get into the competition between our favorite NFL teams, the Dallas Cowboys and the Pittsburgh Steelers. Sam had been a Dallas fan for years and I always liked the Steelers. Today, my son Sam is the Dallas fan and we continue the same rivalry. My son Sam, and my brother Sam would have bonded very well. Each one was and is into knowing what's going on in the sports world, and I mean every sport going.

I believe Sam would have been good in sports. He had that competitive mean streak in him. I was more laid back. Not Sam! Football probably would have been his thing. Sam was Gung Ho more like his Dad. A tough guy all the way around.

One time Sam and I went to our local theater with my friend Val Taylor. It was a terrible day, weather-wise. We went in a blizzard! We were behind a snowplow and couldn't see anything. Sam was very nervous. There was so much snow, Val and I had to pull Sam and his wheelchair through the snow. The movie was terrible and after we got home, we thought, "What were we doing, going out in that kind of weather?" But when you are young and foolish sometimes you have to do those kinds of things. Just another little adventure.

Sam never missed a basketball game while he was in high school. We went to every game even when there was bad weather. Sam was responsible for keeping some stats his senior year. We would have gone to the games regardless. Each gym had its own little spot for Sam and his wheelchair to fit. The first year was a trial by error to find the best spot. Some were good; some weren't so good. From what I can remember, Ludington had the best spot. There was a place at half court between both team benches. Due to the schedule we only played there once a year.

I hate to guess how many trips we made to games. Between regular season and tournaments, there are too many to remember. They were a lot of fun though.

Sam's and My Trip to Florida

In December of 1986, there we were, Sam and I heading to Florida all by ourselves. It was a true adventure! Sam was a little nervous about the trip, always worried about the van breaking down or something going wrong.* But we had a good time together, did a lot of talking. Talked about everything (life in general).

We did have one close call that I will never forget. You know how you can sometimes get into trances, especially on long trips, and not be paying complete attention to what you are doing. We were in Florida (just barely) cruising along about 70 to 75 mph. We were both quiet at this time.

All at once Sam yelled "Tom look out!." I was looking out to the side of road and when I looked ahead of us our lane of traffic was at a dead stop. I swerved left and just missed the car ahead of us. We were both quite rattled. I calmed down right away, but Sam was a nervous

*This was a major undertaking for Tom alone. They spent one night on the road and to do that Tom had to unload the Hoyer Lift, Porta Potty and any other items they might need for the night. Without the above items it would have been almost impossible for any one person to handle Sam alone for a night's stay...

wreak for the rest of the day. He was glad the trip was almost over. All in all we had nice trip together.

After I got married in 1988, Deb, my wife, and I lived in Grand Rapids for a few months. Every Tuesday night was movie night. No matter what! Deb, Sam, I and sometimes Mom would go to the movies. We always hit Studio 28, on 28th street in Grand Rapids, Tuesday night, which was also dollar night. Regular price at that time was around five dollars each. There was always something to watch because at that time there were actually 28 theatres in one building.

That was a good break for the week. It helped the week go faster and gave Sam a chance to get out and get some fresh air. It also gave Mom somewhat of a break. She needed some time to herself once in awhile.

I liked to watch the scary monster type movies . Sam didn't care for them, he always was afraid he would have nightmares. Sam liked the adventure type movies. Deb didn't like either, but she always went. Deb and Sam always got along really well. They liked each other a lot.

One thing that really ticked Sam off, especially at Studio 28, was that the handicapped parking spaces were always filled. We had to drop Sam off then park the van. Sam wanted to give the illegally parked cars a ticket. To park legally in a handicapped parking space you need to have a handicapped sticker on your window or located on your license plate. No one seemed to care about the parking situation and that bothered Sam. But, we kept going to the movies, we had to have our popcorn and soda at least once a week no matter what!

SAM'S OWN WORDS (age 19)

In this section I will talk about four major things: (1) My Life; (2) Camp; (3) The way people react; (4) Love, survival, life, etc.

Throughout the first seven years of my life, I considered my life was just the same as that of any active kid. I really can't recall anything that seemed very difficult for me to do during those first seven years. As I entered third grade, things started changing; things became harder for me to do, especially activities where many muscles had to be used. In fact, my gym teacher was the one who informed my parents that I seemed slower or had more difficulty being active. So the next step was to have a blood test, which turned out positive for muscular dystrophy. The second step was to have a biopsy done, to show what type of dystrophy I had. A biopsy is a little operation where a small piece of muscle is cut so that it can be studied. The test proved that I had "Duchenne" Muscular Dystrophy, and I didn't know it, but my life would never again be the same.

The next two years were probably the toughest years of my life. First, walking became difficult for me.

Because of the problem of balance I walked with or on my toes first; everytime I took a step my toes would hit the ground first. Instead of walking like everybody else I had quite a limp or stagger. Life seemed very cruel to me, not only was I having trouble walking, but many of the other kids teased and made fun of me. There is one incident that really hurt my feelings. I remember it as clearly as if it happened yesterday. It was the last day of school, and I was on my way to the bus after school. As I walked past a bus that was full of high school kids, someone yelled at me, "Hey kid, what's the matter, do you have a stick up your ass or what? I will come down and take it out for you if you say please." Everyone thought that was funnier than hell. That really scares an eight-year-old child; I thought that maybe I was freak or something. I remember when I got home I went to my room and just cried for awhile.

During my ninth year I started falling down every so often, and it happened more and more as time passed. I had to endure great amounts of pain during that year, and by the time I turned ten years old I was ready for a wheelchair. I accepted the fact that a wheelchair was probably the best thing for me. For the first couple of weeks I thought it was great, people lined up to see who would be able to push me at recess and lunch. I almost had to make a schedule or appointment book because everyone wanted to push me. I thought it was great being so popular. I really don't know why everyone was so eager to push me around. Maybe they thought it was cool or they just cared about me and were trying to make me feel better. It was probably a combination of both, but whatever it was, I was grateful for all of it.

However, I soon found out that being in the wheelchair wasn't all that great. After about a month my chauffeurs all liked to go at a fairly good pace, and after a couple of accidents, I became a little frightened. But all of my chauffeurs seemed obsessed with running down the halls, streets, grass, etc. When we started getting older, of course, they started driving safer. After months of me asking them to slow down, they finally were complying with my wishes. Due to all my accidents I came up with bloody noses, cut lips and lumps and scratches. Most of these accidents happened in the fifth grade, my first of being in a wheelchair. There were, however, a couple of these mishaps that were actually quite funny.

Once I tipped over big time, I landed with the pillow I was sitting on underneath my head on the ground. I never did figure out how that could have happened. The other time was in the eighth grade when a couple of girls who were buddies took me for a ride in the school halls. We took a corner pretty fast; they swerved to miss someone and in doing so, we hit a locker and over I went. The books I was carrying were all over the place; we were all laughing on that one.

Also I found that being in a wheelchair was difficult when I saw everyone else walking, playing sports or just goofing around. I was very envious, or better put, felt sorry for myself because I truly loved being active as much as possible. It was very depressing to see people doing things that I could do only a couple of years before.

I counted on people to push me around for six and a half years. I will admit that I was able to push myself somewhat, but it was a tiring and tough job to do. Since everybody wanted to push me, I really didn't have to do it myself very much. I kind of got lazy in that respect. By the time I was in high school I really didn't have the strength to push myself anymore, so I had to totally count on someone to push me anywhere I wanted to go.

By the time I was a 10th grader I decided I'd had enough. I wanted my own wheels so that I could get some of my independence back. So I got an electric wheelchair; this wheelchair became my new legs, so to speak. I got my chair in the spring of 1983 and when I rode into school the next day I was on cloud nine. I had become much more independent in one day's time. I was able to go almost anywhere I wanted to and, believe me, I was a very happy camper. That wheelchair gave me a new lease on life. It still was hard to see everyone else walking and playing sports, but this chair made life more fun for me. For six and a half years, I had gone where others wanted, and stayed there until they left. But now I went where and when I felt like it, and I just loved the idea.

There are times when operations are needed to slow the effects of the disease. In 1980, when I was 13, I had my first entrance into the hospital because of MD. The doctors were going to lengthen my Achille's tendon so that my feet and ankles wouldn't start to curl up due to non-usage. There was a terrible amount of pain after the operation, more than I had anticipated. The pain was terrible and so was the food. It was no fun at all! I had casts on my legs for quite awhile. After a week or two I felt much better. The next thing I had to do was to be fitted for braces to keep the heel cords and feet in the right position. The braces were put on a big black pair of shoes that I really wasn't crazy about. At 13 I was worried about what people would think of my appearance. People say, "Why are you concerned with what people might think?" I'll tell you it doesn't seem like it would be hard, but no one, at any age, wants to be teased or thought of as a freak. I really never was teased or smirked at, but the fear, especially for a 13-year-old, that someone might is a real fear. I think.

As time went by the braces became uncomfortable to wear. They were very hot and sweaty and they started hurting my feet. The pain was too much, and I eventually decided that I would not wear them anymore. To this day I still have some reminders of what the braces did to my feet. My toenails are damaged and a couple of them are almost dead; they made my toes very sensitive to clip, so clipping them is a painful experience. I also have a couple of calluses on the bottom of each foot. All of this was caused by my braces and those black shoes. The operation and braces may have saved by feet for a couple of years, but sometimes I wonder if all the pain, worrying about what people would think, the disappointment and frustration I felt because the operation and braces didn't work was all worth it. My feet started to curl anyway, so really for all practical purposes those days I spent in the hospital were kind of a waste.

February 2, 1984, was probably the saddest day of

my life; my father was dying in the critical care unit of our local hospital. Lung cancer was the villain that had taken my father away from me and my family. About a year before this dreaded day, we had found out that dad had a tumor on his lung. When were told the first thing we thought was, "Oh my God, is he going to die?" The word cancer seemed to mean automatic death; we had been hearing horrible stories about the alarming number of deaths due to this disease. Later we were told that the tumor was in a position where an operation could not be performed to remove it. The tumor had grown very close to his heart and had started wrapping around the heart and lungs and therefore we knew our father was in real trouble.

The next thing was trips my mom and dad had to make to Muskegon, several times per week. My dad had to get radiation treatments and chemical therapy to try to shrink or possibly destroy the cancerous tumor. These treatments made him sick and very tired. It was awful for me and my family to stand by and watch, knowing that there wasn't anything we could do to help him. During the summer of 1983, he was healthy enough to be a base coach for the softball team he had played with for years, in the Class A Finals. He also felt well enough to go deer hunting, which was probably his favorite thing to do, but after that he was pretty much in bed over the next couple of months. I remember New Year's Eve my dad wasn't feeling very good; however, many of his friends stopped in and had a drink. They all wanted to say "hi" and see how he was doing; everyone really showed they cared. It was probably the first New Year's eve in years when he wasn't able to go out and party with his friends. Although he didn't feel good, I think that his friends stopping by made him happy.

About a month later he had to enter our hospital in Ludington, where he was diagnosed with pneumonia and that along with the cancer meant serious problems. The pneumonia weakened my dad, and the cancer was starting to grow again. We all went to visit him on a Wednesday night February 1, 1984, and what we saw scared us. He had oxygen tubes in his nose and he didn't like them and kept taking them out. He was fading in and out of consciousness like he was going to pass out because of lack of air. He would talk for awhile then drift off; it was scary for us. We knew that death couldn't be far off. The next day I got a message that I was going to be picked up at school because of a development with Dad. I just thought he was being transferred to Muskegon, but when they picked me up I was told he had taken a bad turn. While transferring him to Muskegon he had a cardiac arrest, and they had to bring him back to our local hospital. When I got to the hospital, my dad was in a coma and was hooked to some machines. A few minutes after my family and I arrived, the doctors came into the waiting room. They told us that we had to make a decision. We had to decide whether or not to put Dad on life support. Our decision was quick; we all knew that Dad would hate the idea of being kept alive by a machine. So there was no way anyone of us was going to say put him on life support; that is just prolonging death. We believed he had suffered enough already, and so our decision was an easy one. I went into his room with my mom, and I saw all of those machines, the ventilator helping him breathe and the way he was struggling for every breath. It scared me.

You hear doctors say that patients in a coma may be able to hear people, that the hearing is the last to go. Well, I believe it now. My mom was telling Dad that she loved him and that his whole family was there. I swear he moved his head, kind of tilted towards Mom. Anyway, to say the least, it startled me and Mom. After a few more minutes I had to get out of there because I just couldn't stand to see him like that. I knew that it was just a matter of hours before this ordeal would be over. I would only have one parent - it was not easy to take. I could never build enough courage to go back into see him, and after eight hours his heart couldn't take it anymore. He was working so hard to breathe that his heart just gave out. My mom said that it was a very quiet death; there was no struggling, so that made me feel a little better.

My family and I felt a sense of relief; Dad was done suffering and he was going to be in a better place. It was still a shock to realize that you have lost a father. He had lasted a year since the tumor had been discovered. Two days later we had the showing for family and friends and that was a difficult ordeal, seeing my father lying there. He had helped raise me for 16 years; he was gone and it was hard to believe. People came to see and when those people teared up, it made me sad inside. Then Sunday came along, the day of the funeral and that was very sad also. I really didn't cry that much, I guess because there was a time coming, I felt that now I had two diseases to fight, MD and Cancer. The funeral home was just packed - upstairs, downstairs and even outside - just loaded with people. That made me feel great; my pride was overflowing. All of those people came to see my dad; it showed that we had a great father and many people loved and respected him. Many people at the funeral home said that they had never seen so many people at a funeral before.

Our family had gone through a major ordeal and had survived with flying colors. My mom now had many decisions to make; such as getting a better job, moving and just adjusting to life as a single parent; it was a tough time for us. But, we knew that life goes on and that we must stick together and make a new beginning as the Bayles - One for all and all for one.

During the summer of 1984, I found out I had to have another operation that was much more serious. This surgery was one that could add some years to my life, so I almost had to have it. My spine had curved badly over the years of sitting in a wheelchair, and if something wasn't done this would eventually put pressure on my lungs and cause breathing difficulties. When I was told I needed surgery, I just started to cry. I'd known that I would need it someday, but when they told me I needed it sooner than I had expected I became scared. Luckily I had a talk with someone else who had had the same operation a few months earlier. He told me that he had been scared too, and that the operation had helped him a lot. He made me feel a little bit more at ease, but I was still very frightened. I had to do a lot of thinking about whether or not to have the operation, which meant taking a huge risk or having the surgery and maybe adding years to my life. I even was afraid that I might not make it; maybe I would die on the table. So many thoughts were running through my head, but in the long run it was no contest; I had to have it done. The doctors were going to put metal bars, one on each side of my spine. This operation took about six hours, and I needed a blood transfusion, so it was quite a major task.

When I woke up I was one scared 17-year-old kid, there were tubes and machines all over me. Something was helping me to breathe, with tubes in my nose and throat. I tried to fight it because I could breathe on my own, and everytime I tried beepers and a light flashed. Those scared me also, but finally I accepted what was going on and things settled down a bit. I told myself to be positive and that I was going to recover and get out of the hospital as soon as possible. As each day came I looked forward to another tube being removed, and three days later I was moved out of intensive care to a regular room, and after three more days I was able to leave the hospital and head home. In fact, I surprised the doctors by recovering so quickly that I was able to leave the hospital before they had expected me to.

Then when I got home I had a bed set up in the living room so that I could recover the rest of the way, with all of the comforts of home. I also had to readjust to being in an upright position with a straight back; all of my movements had to be modified because of my straight back. It was kind of like learning to walk again, and it was a challenge that I would win. After about three weeks I felt up to going back to school, and when I did it felt like a new beginning of the new, improved Sam Bayle was unleashed into the world to begin his senior year. This operation was going to keep my lungs clearer and more open, so that I would be able to help fight colds easier. Colds were a major enemy that I must be able to fight off. If my lungs were not clear, the chance of getting pneumonia or bad congestion would threaten my health.

Many of my best memories were my years at Mason County Central. Probably my two happiest or proudest moments were graduation and having the yearbook dedicated to me. Graduation meant a lot to me because I know there are some people with MD who never make it. Being able to graduate with some of the nicest people I will ever be associated with was a great honor, an accomplishment for me, and it is very hard to explain. I just felt great. The yearbook was a surprise to me; I didn't ever have a hint of something that great. It meant that my classmates really cared for me a tremendous amount, and there is not a better feeling in the world. I mean, with that many friends there is hardly a challenge that will stop me. Also the speech that my mom gave was a total shock. I had no idea she had something up her sleeve. But the things she said were all true, that I really appreciated the help my classmates gave me through the years which helped me a lot. I probably would or should have said those things to my classmates, but I would have gotten too emotional and would have given a terrible speech. Anyway, I love

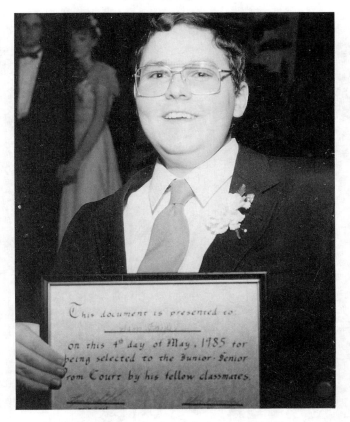

Sam after being inducted into the National Honor Society.

everyone of my classmates for the way they willingly helped me get along and made my high school years ones I will never forget.

There are three other things that I felt good about in high school. The first is that I had a chance to do basketball stats for three years. I really enjoyed following the basketball team, and doing the stats made me a little part of the team. Another important thing was when I got my school letter for sports because I did stats. Since I couldn't play sports, having a letter meant a lot and I wore it with

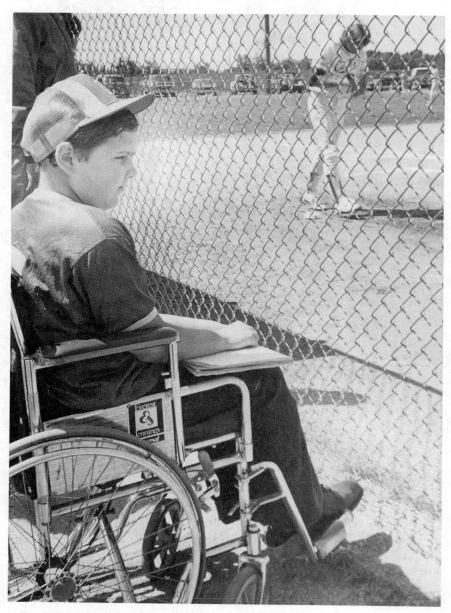

Official statistician for dad's softball team.

pride. I enjoyed being inducted as an honorary member of the National Honor Society in a special induction for someone who displays courage or leadership and may set a good standard for people to follow. This was a great honor for me because this meant that people thought I displayed these good qualities.

The other two things happened on the end of Spirit Week (homecoming week) on a Friday when all of the classes battle each other to see who is best. When I was a junior, the judges let me race my wheelchair against the rest of the school. It was kind of neat to see everyone go nuts when I had a brief lead over the seniors. At the beginning of the race when I was a senior, I got to lead our class into the gym pulling three wagons and blowing a whistle like a train. The look of amazement and interest on everybody's face was fun, and we came home with first place in the spirit week challenge.

Many of my other achievements have taken place in the sport of amateur softball. In the summer of 1984, I set up and ran the Custer VFW tourney the tournament that my dad had run for nine years until he passed away in February of 1984. It was quite a challenge for me, but in the long run the tournament turned out to be one of the best ever. The VFW post had changed the tournament name to the Howard Bayle Memorial, and the tournament was a great success. This made me very proud of myself and also of the tourney named in memory of my father.

Also, in 1984, I took the job of handling the county softball stats for 40 plus teams, and that was a tremendous job. But I did probably as well as anybody had done in the past. With the help of my mom, I came up with a plan for compiling and reporting the stats. We were able to print all softball stats in the local newspaper three times instead of the usual one time per summer. This also made me proud of myself.

In the summer of 1985, I was asked to coach a softball team, which included some of my friends. Being a coach had always been one of my dreams and all of a sudden I was. In the first season the team compiled a record of 10 wins and 10 losses. The season was a challenge for me; the players had trouble getting to the games on time. I felt that the team didn't listen to me as much as I had hoped, but that wasn't all of their fault either; it was my first year as a coach and I just was not as assertive as I could have been. Also, the sponsor usually made most of the decisions, and though again that was partly my fault, I felt as if I didn't have a chance to really show what I could do. We did win our league title that year and played pretty well in the state district tournament before blowing out. But all and all with the minimum of players we had a good year. The next year I only coached five games, but the team showed signs of improvement even though their record was 2-3. But the last game I coached the team played probably one of the best games in my coaching career in a higher league. Even though their record was 2-3 when I left, they went on to win the districts, regionals and ended with a sixth place finish in the state finals with a 21-14 record. My career was 12-13, and I didn't think that was too bad. Although I realized if I was ever going to be a good coach, I was going to have to become more assertive and do what I think is right and feel very positive about it. Coaching my friends in softball was a good learning experience for me in future projects.

MUSCULAR DYSTROPHY SUMMER CAMP: The key words here are **LOVE** and **FRIENDSHIP**. I have gone to camp for 10 years now, and it seems to get better each year and the word love comes to my mind, perhaps because love was so abundant there. At the age of 10, when Mom left the camp, I cried because it was really the first time I had been away from home. It took me only a half an hour to get over that, then I was having a great time. I also remember that when it was time to go home, I cried again. I cried all day when I got home because I missed my counselor and friends. It is quite amazing how close you can become to your counselor in just one week.

When someone spends 24 hours a day with someone, learning how to care for their campers, I guess my reaction really isn't surprising. I can say from experience that the first couple of hours are very important for a counselor and camper to get to know each other. I think it is important to ask your helper what he expects and then kind of fill him or her in on things that they will need to know and do to help out. Patience is another very important aspect that in my opinion a camper must have. I know that each counselor I've had was very nervous hoping their camper will like them; they were also afraid that they wouldn't do things correctly.

Many counselors really don't know what to expect. So the first couple of days a camper should take them through step by step so that they can learn every thing correctly. After three or four days it is like they have been helping you for years. So there is really no reason to be afraid to ask them for anything.

There is one thing that does bother me; that's when a camper makes their counselor cry because of a bad attitude or because they don't care for their attendant. I mean it ruins not only your attendant's week, but in the long run yours too. I can say that in my ten years I've liked all my counselors; there were a couple who weren't what I call my favorite kind of person, but there were things I liked about them and we had a good time. These people are there to help you, so there is no reason to wreck your whole week. The volunteers who help take care of the campers are very special people. They come to camp because they care for others just as much or more than themselves.

Camp gives campers a week to feel free to try new things like dancing, bowling, swimming and playing cards and many other games. Dancing is a lot of fun moving as much as you can; girls will hold your hand. Some of the girls will sit on the arm rest of the wheelchair or on your lap, or get on their knees and hug you like during a slow dance. It is something I really enjoy because I never had a chance while I was walking. I probably could go to a dance place, but I would most likely be the only one in a wheelchair. Everyone would stare and have their own date; it just is not the same. Going swimming is something I used to love to do; I'm sure that most of the campers don't get a chance to swim during the rest of the year. People will go into the pool to help get you in and take you around the pool; you will have a life jacket on and going into the pool is fun. Personally, I don't mind swimming, but I find that by the time I get my suit and life jacket on, that accompanied with not being able to stay up on my legs, it just is not worth it. Because of the disease I am not strong enough to stay upright; the life jacket floats so I just fall on my back.

Since I am such a free spirit, I don't like to be completely dependent on someone while playing sports. Hockey, bowling and whiffle ball are just a tremendous amount of fun. I've always loved sports, but was never able to play. In hockey each person gets a hockey stick and we go after it; sometimes we will have wheelchair accidents around the puck, but it is a lot of fun. As far as bowling, we are not able to throw the ball so we use a little ramp. We line the ball up to where we think it will be a strike, and we push it down the ramp. Whiffle ball is a game in which counselors play a big part. The campers who can swing a bat do, and those who can't, get help from their attendant. Someone pitches the ball and the campers hit it. Then, depending on the kind of chair they have, the campers either drive themselves or their counselor pushes them around the bases. Probably the thing I enjoy most is visiting with friends, playing games like cards, checkers or a variety of others and listening to music. I have many friends, campers, counselors and staff that I see once a year, just during this week annually. It's nice to see and visit with them, to see what they have done over the year or what they plan to do next.

It is really like one big family. There is just a lot of

love being given out and shared between the campers, counselors and every staff member. Being with people who understand what we are going through make us feel like there is nothing wrong. Getting together with others who have MD gives us a chance to discuss our lives and become good friends, and each year we meet in June to have our annual get together. It is just like a great family reunion, and I can say that it is the highlight of my summer, and it would be a big disappointment if I ever had to miss it. It is a place where I feel on top of the world, almost like heaven. It is just a very special place where love and friendship are shared. It also gives our parents a chance to relax from all of the things that they do for us, that we count on them for. It is hard to say good-bye to our counselors at the end of our week.

When you spend 24 hours a day for a week together you can't help but become good friends. These counselors come to camp as volunteers, to help the campers enjoy a week of freedom and the chance to try new things and just have a great time doing it. I have a tremendous amount of respect and admiration for each and every one of these caring people. You know, if it wasn't for the disease, I would have never met any of these people. The idea of not ever having met these people is just not a good thought. I can also say that some of my best friends were at camp. Over the past ten years counting all of my friends in my head is difficult. Sometimes you might never see these people again, but you know that you have a friend out there somewhere if you need them. Camp is the highlight of my summer, and I know 65 other campers who will

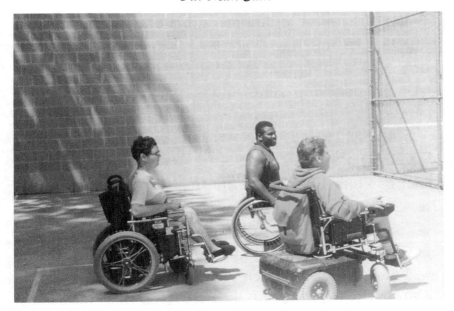

A wheelchair basketball game at camp.

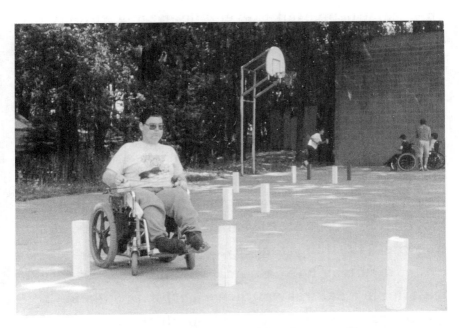

A race against time through the cones. "Don't knock any over!"

agree; it is the most loving place that I know. It is a lot of fun to keep in touch with some of the people throughout the year by writing letters or talking on the phone, until next summer - camp comes and you can reunite with your friends.

BEING TREATED AS AN EQUAL: Not being treated as an equal is a major point of frustration for me. People sometimes talk differently to me than they might to anyone else. They probably don't even realize it, but it is there. They act as if they have to spare me some details that may hurt my ears concerning girls, drinking or other things that I may not do as much. Sometimes when I'm with a couple of friends, they will start a conservation and almost ignore me completely. Also people feel they have to treat me special, and I know it is just because I'm in a wheelchair. These same people talk to everyone else much differently, and again they probably don't realize it. All I want is to be treated the same as anyone else; I'm the same as any other guy, only I have wheels instead of legs.

GIRLS: Girls are another major area of frustration for me. This is very hard to talk about, but I'm going to give it a try. Girls seem hesitant or a little afraid to talk to me. I believe many see the wheelchair and for some reason talk to me differently than they would otherwise. Maybe it is because they realize that I may not be able to do some of the things that guys who walk can. To a certain extent they may have a point; after all, I can't dance, at least not in a natural way, drive a car to pick them up, or go for walks on the beach. Also, there are many little things I need help with. I feel that I have just as much or more to offer than any other guy.

Many of my friends who are also wheelchair bound say that girls they meet always want to be just friends and nothing more. That's fine for awhile, but after a few girls it gets to be an old story because we start to wonder whether it is just because we are in wheelchairs. Will we ever get a chance to have a close relationship in our lives? In the last six to eight years there are many girls I would have liked to have known better, but I felt a sense of insecurity or hesitancy from them. I also felt: why should I put any girls through a night where they might not have as much fun with me as they would with a walker? But, afterwards I would kick myself for not asking some of the girls to be my girl, because I have a tremendous amount of good things to give and would enjoy receiving. All I want is an equal opportunity to show a girl what I can share with her; after all I'm the same as any other guy; I have emotions, I can talk and I'm fun to be with.

As I get older, I'm envious of other couples having fun together. When guys treat their girls in a bad way, I say to myself "If I was more confident, and was given an equal chance I could be a good partner". Even at summer camp the girls treat or talk and act to us much differently than to anyone else. They act real cozy and flirty with walkers and treat us like little kids, when in reality I am, or we are, usually older than the counselors. We are not aliens, apes, or little babies, we are normal guys and gals except we have a disease called MD. I am a real good friend, but I really wish I could have a girl in my life.

There are two major circumstances, for me, that I

believe keep a relationship from happening. My confidence is one, I'm afraid of what a girl's answer might be. I think that all would say no because of my wheelchair. I would like to have a chance to walk for a couple of weeks and see if I could go out with a girl and become more than friends with her. This would prove my suspicions. The other factor that stops me is I get the feeling some think they might be able to catch MD. I realize that it would take a very special girl to see past the chair and want more than friendship. There are many things I can't do as compared to a walker, but there are many things in life to share with someone special that wouldn't include whether or not I could walk. Sharing my life with someone special is an important part of my future. Girls just don't think we have as much to offer as guys who can walk. With a little help from a girl I can dance close, make out, hug!! Driving is a little difficult, but with a little imagination and patience, everything can be fun.

I was 20 years old before I had a date; a lot of it was a lack of confidence. A couple girls I asked to go with me as a boyfriend; they said no, but then a couple days later they were going with another guy. It was a real slap in the face. You see, they said they didn't want a relationship at this time, but two days later they were going with someone else. This really destroyed my confidence. Maybe I was wrong, but the first thing I thought is that it was because of the wheels. Where I live there are only a couple of places to go on a date, to a dance or to a movie. As for a dance place, I wasn't the type of person to go and be the only one in a wheelchair and dance differently from other people. I really wouldn't want to put my girl through that. She would probably get all kinds of questions from her girlfriends and other peers, and I didn't want to put that kind of pressure on anyone. During my high school years I went without a relationship or a date. I really wish I knew why girls acted like I was a fragile person. This may be out in left field, but maybe girls feel better when a guy is the one in charge. Maybe girls are afraid to control things such as driving, helping me and not being able to have me care for them, without their help.

When I met someone who treated me as an equal, I fell into a trap where I wanted a relationship so badly I tried to rush things. One girl I fell in love with, but she wanted to be just friends. That was fine, but it gets to be an old story. I have had many female friends, but I would like to have a girlfriend someday. I just haven't found the right girl yet. I know it is going to take a special person who is very caring inside. I think this person is out there somewhere, but I hope I'm able to find her soon. In the back of our minds we are all scared that we may never have a feeling of being loved. We are afraid that we might miss out on one of the best things in life, a close relationship with someone of the opposite sex. We are also afraid that we might not ever be able to show someone what we can give them. Love and friendship are ready to be shared.

BEING INDEPENDENT: This is something I will have to live with, but sometimes it can get me down and upset because of the many things I cannot do without help. From putting on my clothes to eating, bathing, going to the bathroom, making dinner and driving.

Knowing that I count on people for many things and that without them I am up a creek is just hard for me to take because I have such an active spirit. This is one of the reasons I love my electric wheelchair so much because I can go many places by myself. If someone sighs or complains that they have to do something for me, it makes me mad and sad. However, I can see where they are coming from, because I do need a lot of care every day and it can become very tiring. Whatever I can do for myself and my independence makes me happy.

SPORTS: Sports have been a major part of my life for as long as I can remember. Many of my dreams involved the sports world, and everytime I see someone playing basketball, football, baseball, golf it makes me cringe and I wish I could do the same. Now, I try to do whatever I can to be involved in sports - coaching, keeping stats, being a good fan, reading magazines or just watching them. It is not what I wish it could be, but that is just something I'm going to have to live with. I've dreamed of making a winning basket or a homerun or great catch to make my team a winner. I used to become upset and cry, when I was younger, when kids left me to play some sport. It will always be a tender spot for me, and I'll just have to be involved in sports as much as possible.

There are some advantages to being in a wheelchair. Things such as parking, seats and just courteous people who let me do things. As far as parking, there are special places usually near the entrance to stores, ball parks or just about any place. At the Pontiac Silverdome we got to park right near an entrance, drive up to the front door essentially. Seating is another perk that involves wheelchairs. At most professional sport parks, they have special places for wheelchairs, with an excellent viewing section. Another example of special treatment I remember was in Washington D.C. The parking was great for vehicles carrying wheelchairs at the monuments and the White House. During my high school career there was a lady who made my hot lunch for me daily. Things like that are neat for wheelchair bound people.

Softball has been a major part of my life for years. I watched my dad, brother and friends play softball each

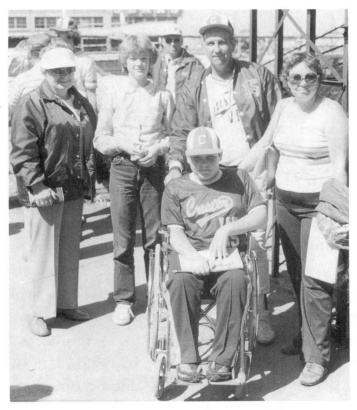

Waiting for the next tournament game with Grandma Bayle, Stacy, Dad and Mom.

and every summer for as long as I can remember. In the town and county where I lived for 19 years, softball is a big activity that involves a lot of people in one way or another. My dad played for a long time and when he went out of town to play, the whole family went along. Mom and I were great fans, and my brother and sister played games with the other kids at the ballpark. We were definitely a softball family. My brother started playing and I kept stats for a couple of teams and eventually for the whole county. I became a coach for one year and part of another and softball was just a large part of our lives. We followed my dad's and brother's team very closely for years and even though we moved, we still kept in touch and saw as many games as possible.

During my life my family and I have taken two trips, one to Wyoming and one to Washington D.C. My dad was still around when we took the trip out west. We took in museums, zoos and many other exhibits, the countryside was breathtaking and very exciting. My dad and a few other guys used to go out to Wyoming to hunt Mule Deer and Antelope. We went to a ranch where they went hunting, and we got to explore the many acres of this beautiful ranch. It was neat. This was the last year that I was able to walk a little. We had taken a wheelchair because I was starting to have problems walking. This trip lasted about ten days and it was an interesting and learning experience. It will be a trip that I'll never forget and something I think everyone should do.

After my dad died, my family and I went to Washington, D.C. We saw all of the monuments, the

White House and Mount Vernon. We learned a lot of American history, and we went to as many museums and history exhibits as we could. I got to see the Phillies play the Pittsburgh Pirates at Three Rivers Stadium in Pittsburgh. The Phillies won the game, and I just loved it. We went to Hershey Park, Chocolate Capital of the world. We had a tour of the factory and toured the park in a major downpour, but we had fun anyway. This trip lasted about a week, and we had a great time; it was nice getaway for us.

COURAGE: Courage is something that is important to survival, not just for people with MD, but for everyone who has problems. Courage, to me, means the ability to stand and face problems with the attitude of positive thinking, to make problems into good things instead of letting your problems grow and control your life. I think that people who think and commit suicide start to let their problems control their lives and they can see no way out except to jump. People think I have a lot of courage and they are right to an extent. I have usually one bad day every two weeks where I feel sorry for myself, but my courage takes me out of those moods. I face up to the fact that I have problems, but there are many more people with problems much greater than mine who face up to them and overcome them. But I am a free spirit. I start to feel bad because of something I can't do, or if I see couples having a good time together or little things that I can't even understand why. I get a feeling of helplessness because of things I cannot do, having to count on someone all of the time for everything that I might need. I get a closed-in feeling and become depressed. There are also times when I feel I'm getting weaker because of the disease. This leads me to fearing what will happen in my future years. This fear concerns even my ability to eat, brush my teeth and play games by myself. I don't want to have to give up even these easy to do things and become totally dependent on someone else. I see many people at camp who need this kind of care and they still smile, so maybe my fear is selfish. Being unable to do certain things that others can is just something I must live with. As far as those couples go, it bothers me to see them, mainly because I'm envious. These two things are what trigger my bad spells, but they only last a couple of hours. I'm sure many people have this same "feeling sorry for yourself syndrome," and I think courage can help bring you out of these moods. There are some people who couldn't and can't handle having MD or other similar problems and there are people who kill themselves even though they seem to have everything you could want. Courage is within everyone; it is just whether or not you can reach inside yourself and find it.

JERRY LEWIS TELETHON: These telethons are very important to all of the people who have a neuromuscular disease. The money raised helps those people live life as easily as possible. Without the money I would have no electric wheelchair or any chair at all. That would take all of my independence away, and life would be miserable without it. Money provides things that slow the progress of the disease, such as braces, chairs or lifts. Many of the dollars go for research trying to find out what causes MD and to find a cure to wipe it out. In 1986, the research team found the faulty gene that causes MD; now they must find out what makes this gene become irregular and why it is so destructive. The finding of this gene is a major discovery and it gives all people with MD a glimmer of hope that someday a cure will be found. The scientists now know where to concentrate their work and I'm confident they will find the cure very soon. The cure may not be found soon enough to help me, but if it can stop other people from getting it, nothing would be more satisfying or make me happier. I would not wish this disease on my worst enemy, so I will be happy for others and not feel sorry for myself.

Jerry Lewis is a man who is made of gold both inside and out. He has dedicated his life to the cause of MD and will be involved until his death. There is no person I would rather meet in this whole world. He has raised millions of dollars for MD, and he loves every one of his "Kids". His heart is just chock full of love. If there were more people like him in the world, the earth would be a much safer and better place to live. If everyone in the U.S. put one dollar towards the MD Telethon, it would raise 250 million dollars, about as much as the telethon makes in eight years. One dollar is not much for any one person to use wisely, and I know you would be feeling proud of yourself for doing it. I know the cry for money gets tiresome, but every cent you give helps someone have a better life. I have been able to be part of a few telethons over the years.

Another experience I probably wouldn't have had if it weren't for the disease is my exposure on television. I have been on TV three or four times and really consider it a privilege to have had this chance. It is a neat feeling to be on TV; but knowing that there are a lot of people watching makes it nerve racking. When it is live, there is no way you can change how you look or what you say. Taping my appearances is something that is fun because you can watch it over many times, and you can show people who are interested . I was proud to be on TV, I'm not sure why, but I guess it is something not every one gets a chance to do. I might get people to give more and that might be the thing that helps scientists get over the top and find a cure for the 40 neuromuscular diseases that make up the group called Muscular Dystrophy. The cure will soon be found!

MY ONE BIG REGRET
AS A PARENT

Through Sam's life, we as a family experienced many different things. My one big regret is that I never pursued, hard enough, a dream of Sam's. He wanted one day to meet Jerry Lewis. Sam had the greatest faith that Jerry would be "The Scientist" to discover a cure for Muscular Dystrophy. I tried to explain that Jerry didn't actually do the testing, but made the money so scientists could do the discovering. I know his biggest thrill of a lifetime would have been to meet Jerry Lewis and thank him for his love and support. I don't know if it could have been accomplished, but I wish I had tried harder to make that dream come true. I kept saying to myself, I have time to work on this dream. I waited too long. My thought to other parents, in the same circumstances, don't wait too long to work on a special dream of their child.

FINAL WORDS

I know in my heart they are close to helping the kids with muscular dystrophy, especially Duchenne; don't give up hope that in your child's lifetime there will be a cure. As the doctors are studying Duchenne, they are also learning about the other types of dystrophy. Just remember to live your lives to the fullest; don't be afraid to have dreams and give life your best shot. I believe that we did help Sam lead a full life and that he helped us learn not to feel sorry for yourself; you need to manage the hand you have been dealt to the best of your ability. Everyone has problems and, if you look around you, you will see there is someone with worse problems to live with than yours.

REVIEWING OUR FAMILY'S LIVES SINCE SAM HAS PASSED AWAY

Tom and his wife Debbie have two children; they named their first born son, "Sam." What could be a more fitting tribute? Stacy is married and living in New Mexico, studying to be a Special Ed Teacher. Stacy has always been good with children and with her first-hand experience helping Sam, she will be an excellent candidate to teach Special Ed. I still live in the Scottville area. I work in a school system and because our home was leveled to build a bypass, I have built a new home on the same property. I am involved with a great guy, who has helped me put my life back together again.

For Additional Copies of

Susan Bayle's

S Our Man
Sam

send check or money order for $9.95, plus $3.50 shipping & handling to:

Our Man Sam
424 W. Johnson Road
Scottville, MI 49454

Michigan residents add 6% sales tax, or $.60 for each book.